Nursing Process in
COLLABORATIVE PRACTICE

A Problem-Solving Approach

second edition

Nursing Process in

COLLABORATIVE PRACTICE

A Problem-Solving Approach

second edition

Carol Vestal Allen, PhD, RN, CNAA
Chief, Performance Improvement Service
Department of Veterans Affairs Medical Center
Las Vegas, Nevada

Second Edition

Appleton & Lange
Stamford, Connecticut

Copyright © 1997 by Appleton & Lange
A Simon & Schuster Company

96 97 98 99 00 / 10 9 8 7 6 5 4 3 2 1

Prentice Hall International (UK) Limited, *London*
Prentice Hall of Australia Pty. Limited, *Sydney*
Prentice Hall Canada, Inc., *Toronto*
Prentice Hall Hispanoamericana, S.A., *Mexico*
Prentice Hall of India Private Limited, *New Delhi*
Prentice Hall of Japan, Inc., *Tokyo*
Simon & Schuster Asia Pte. Ltd., *Singapore*
Editora Prentice Hall do Brasil Ltda., *Rio de Janeiro*
Prentice Hall, *Upper Saddle River, New Jersey*

Library of Congress Cataloging-in-Publication Data

Allen, Carol Vestal.
    Nursing process in collaborative practice : a problem-solving
approach / Carol Vestal Allen.
        p. cm.
    Rev. ed. of: Comprehending the nursing process. c1991.
    Includes bibliographical references and index.
    ISBN 0–8385–1467–7 (pbk. : alk. paper)
    1. Nursing—Case studies. 2. Health care teams—Case studies.
I. Allen, Carol Vestal   Comprehending the nursing process.
II. Title
    [DNLM: 1. Nursing Process—organization & administration—
examination questions. 2. Managed Care Programs—examination
questions. 3. Patient Care Planning—examination questions. WY
18.2 A425n   1996]
RT41.A43   1996
610.73—dc20
DNLM/DLC
for Library of Congress   96–8018
                                                        CIP

Acquisitions Editor: David Carroll
Development Editor: Barbara Severs
Production Editor: Maria T. Vlasak
Designer: Mary Skudlarek

PRINTED IN THE UNITED STATES OF AMERICA

REVIEWERS

Marjorie Allen, MA
Instructor, Interlink at
Valparaiso University
Valparaiso, Indiana

Katherine Johnson Bradley, MSN, RN
Doctoral Candidate, Instructional Technology,
Wayne State University
Assistant Director of the Nursing Program
Wayne County Community College
Detroit, Michigan
Commander, Nurse Corps,
United States Naval Reserve
Former Head, Reserve Medical Education
and Training
Naval Health Sciences Education
and Training Command
Bethesda, Maryland

Janice Coleman, MSN, RN, CNS
Associate Professor of Nursing
Jefferson Community College
Louisville, Kentucky

Ann L. Lambeth, MS, RN
Mesa State College
Nursing and Allied Health
Grand Junction, Colorado

Joann Pieronek, PhD, RN
Director of the Nursing Program
Wayne County Community College
Former Dean, Division of Nursing
Mercy College of Detroit
Detroit, Michigan

Mary Ellen Smith, MSN, RN, CS
Assistant Professor
Hahnemann University, School of Health Sciences
and Humanities
Philadelphia, Pennsylvania

CONTENTS

FOREWORD

The current changes in health care focus on decreasing the cost of care, shortening inpatient hospital stays, shifting practice from hospital inpatient units to outpatient clinics and community settings, and creating non-professional health care provider roles. During this time of change, it is imperative for the nursing profession to capture and measure nursing's unique contribution to client care, while at the same time, to adhere to professional standards of conduct and performance. The delivery of the same level of competent care must be ensured in the health care system. The nursing process, a problem-solving method, provides a common framework to facilitate the structure, process, and outcome operations undertaken by nursing staff and an interdisciplinary team.

The textbook *Nursing Process in Collaborative Practice* emphasizes the changes in health care and implementation of the problem-solving approach by nurses and the interdisciplinary health care team. Carol Allen has experience in teaching nursing staff and interdisciplinary team members to assist clients through a continuum of care, in conducting interdisciplinary assessment of clients, and in managing interdisciplinary client and family teaching. The present changes in health care delivery provide the nursing profession with an opportunity to assume a major role in case management, ensuring that the health care needs of diverse clients are met.

The author brings to this project successful experience teaching the nursing process to nursing students and nursing staff. She conducted a multisite research study on *The Effect of Inservice Education Concerning the Nursing Process on Motivating Registered Nurses to Change Their Behavior Toward Implementation of the Nursing Process in Medical Centers.* As a member of two People-to-People Nursing Delegations, to the Far East and Eastern Europe, she led panels and scientific exchanges on the nursing process, bringing clarity to the understanding of this concept to our professional nursing counterparts abroad. *Nursing Process in Collaborative Practice* reflects the shift of health care into an interdisciplinary collaborative practice model and represents in the written medium much of Carol Allen's clinical experience, research, and teachings, which can be of benefit to many nursing students, nursing clinicians, and interdisciplinary health care team members.

Gertrude K. McFarland, DNSc, RN, FAAN
Health Scientist Administrator
Nursing Research Study Section, Division
    of Research Grants
National Institutes of Health
US Department of Health and Human Services
Bethesda, Maryland

PREFACE

Nursing Process in Collaborative Practice, embraces the changes that are occurring in health care, specifically the thrust into an interdisciplinary delivery of care. The title of the first edition, *Comprehending the Nursing Process* (1991), has been changed to reflect current trends in health care practice. The interdisciplinary team consists of health care providers from such disciplines as nursing, medicine, pharmacy, dietetics, physical therapy, occupational therapy, recreational therapy, psychology, social work, and chaplaincy. Team members work together in caring for clients with health problems that are multiple and more complex than those in the past. The team also faces challenges other than complex health problems. For example, the workload of the team is increasing as a result of the cutbacks in health services. In addition, team members represent different backgrounds, abilities, and knowledge bases.

The problem-solving approach provides the team members with a systematic approach to client care and a common professional language and facilitates the delivery of the same level of competent care to all clients.

Nursing Process in Collaborative Practice is designed for independent self-paced or classroom learning by nursing students, faculty, and clinicians. The text describes current trends in health care and the influence of change on the delivery of care. The new chapters in the second edition include information on providing a continuum of care, the initiation of case management, primary care, clinical pathways, clinical practice guidelines, and the role of computers in facilitating the transmission of information. The book emphasizes the incorporation of the problem-solving approach into all aspects of care. Interdisciplinary plans of care, clinical practice guidelines, and nursing care plans are similar in that the problem-solving approach is used to assess the client, identify the priority problem(s), establish a plan of action and expected outcomes, implement the plan, and evaluate the effectiveness of the plan in achieving the outcomes.

Thinking logically in the face of turmoil is an ability required of the interdisciplinary team members. The increased threat of malpractice looms over clinicians. Avoiding judgment errors is essential. The problem-solving approach is a valuable tool for nurses and other team members. The nurse and the interdisciplinary team weigh the priorities of care and decide on a course of action. With the increase in the cost of care and in the cost of health insurance, clients want their "money's worth" and demand the achievement of desired outcomes at minimal cost. Coordination of care by the interdisciplinary team is essential and may lead to a reduction in the cost of care. Interdisciplinary plans of care incorporate components previously found on nursing care plans. Nurses need to collaborate with other disciplines in coordinating the clients' care by using the problem-solving approach in thinking through solutions.

The content in the second edition is presented in a clear succinct manner. The book is targeted primarily to student nurses. Mini case studies, threaded throughout the textbook, illustrate the content, and applicable exercises follow each step of the problem-solving approach. Answers are provided for all of the exercises. Two major case studies further facilitate application of content. In Chapter 8, a medical case study is presented using Gordon's Functional Health Patterns as the assessment framework. In Chapter 9, a surgical case study is presented using a modified body-systems approach as the assessment model. Functional Health Patterns and a body-systems approach may be used by interdisciplinary teams.

Throughout the book, the word *client* refers to the individual, family, significant other, or the community. The word *family* is used to designate individuals who are significant to the client. Family includes an individual(s) who may or may not be legally related to the client. The term, *outcome* is synonymous with client goals, objectives, expected outcomes, outcome behaviors, or short- and long-term goals. Each phase of the problem-solving process is explained in the textbook and followed by an exercise. The exercises assist learn-ers to become actively involved in the application of the phases of problem solving and in developing critical thinking abilities.

The information provided in the textbook applies to all areas of health care including nursing. For example, the information helps nurses who practice in medical-surgical, maternal and newborn, pediatric, psychiatric-mental health, community health, critical care, emergency, ambulatory care, physicians' office, and long-term care settings.

Threading the problem-solving approach consistently throughout a curriculum or health care setting ensures continuity of learning and facilitates the delivery of consistent, competent care. Readers have uniformly cited the up-to-date information and practical details presented as the feature that sets *The Nursing Process in Collaborative Practice* apart from other textbooks.

Carol Vestal Allen

ACKNOWLEDGMENTS

A special thank you to my children, Marjorie and Peter, for their steadfast support throughout this project and all my endeavors.

I wish to acknowledge the staff at Appleton & Lange who contributed to the textbook, especially Barbara Severs, who offered concrete suggestions and supported the changes in the second edition that were based on current trends in health care. She was diligent and detailed in her editing and clarifying of the content.

I am grateful to Dr. Gertrude McFarland for writing a thought-provoking Foreword.

Propelling the Delivery of Health Care into the 21st Century

Customers (clients, patients, families) demand satisfaction with health care services. They want programs that promote wellness and services that resolve identified health problems or concerns. Customers demand to know the names of health care organizations that achieve the best outcomes of care and the greatest results for the amount of money charged for services. Accrediting bodies such as the Joint Commission of Accreditation of Healthcare Organizations (JCAHO) conduct surveys and publish the results for public scrutiny. Therefore, consumers will possess knowledge of health care providers who consistently meet established standards and achieve expected outcomes. Health care providers are compelled to define their practice in measurable terms. This permits the consumers to make informed decisions in the selection of health care providers.

The enormity of these changes brings forth new challenges to all health care disciplines. For example, what is the unique measurable contribution of nursing in meeting the customers' needs and effecting cost saving measures? Changes have been initiated in the health care system to meet the customers' needs, stimulate competition among health care agencies, and curb the increase in health care costs. Major stimuli for change stem from several factors:

- the US government's Agenda for Health Care Reform
- the JCAHO shift to the measurement of continuous performance improvement
- the Agency for Health Care Policy and Research's (AHCPR) dissemination of clinical practice guidelines

- the American Nurses Association's (ANA) Standards of Clinical Nursing Practice (see Appendix K).

All of the above agencies focus on the achievement of measurable client outcomes through the delivery of effective (measured by outcomes achieved) and efficient (cost-saving) care. The care may be delivered at inpatient and outpatient facilities, in the clients' homes, and long-term care settings.

The US government's Agenda for Health Care Reform calls for collaboration among health care facilities to develop strategies to deliver cost-effective and efficient care accessible to all citizens. The government plans to develop tactics for providing universal health care coverage to all citizens in addition to containing the growth of health care cost. Universal access to health insurance would alleviate the burden placed on health care facilities to absorb the cost of care rendered to uninsured clients.

Health care costs could be reduced by emphasizing primary and preventive care, full immunizations, prenatal care, healthier life-styles, and client participation in the economic consequences of their health care decisions. Population-specific health promotion and disease prevention programs play an increasingly important role in reducing medical care costs. The nursing profession has an opportunity to claim a niche in the preventive aspect of health care.

Leadership from the nursing profession and other health care professions is essential in accomplishing health care reform and to set the nation on a path of sustained improvement in health. The changes that are occurring offer nursing an opportunity to improve the profession's contribution to the health and well-being of the population. Initiating incremental health care reforms will be more effective than sweeping changes that lead to turmoil and uncertainty.

■ DELIVERING CONSISTENT, COMPETENT CARE

Leaders of health care organizations design strategies to ensure the uniform delivery of client care throughout an organization. Clients with the same health problems have a right to receive the same level of competent care. For example, clients with the same nursing care needs receive a comparable level of competent nursing care throughout an organization; the care does not differ from shift to shift or from nurse to nurse. For example, clients receiving intravenous conscious sedation (diazepam [Valium]) resulting in the loss of protective reflexes (swallowing) receive the same level of care whether the clients are in the operating room, dental service, endoscopy or bronchoscopy room, and the staff providing the care demonstrate the same competency (expertise). Standards, clinical practice guidelines, and clinical pathways help ensure the delivery of consistent, competent care.

Standards

Standards help to ensure a consistent level of competent care for clients entering a health care system. Standards are generally accepted criteria by which things of the same class are compared in order to determine quantity or excellence. For example, specific standards are used to determine whether clients receive from all nurses the same standard of care in an intensive care unit.

JCAHO's Standards. The JCAHO is an independent body that accredits health care organizations on the basis of established standards of health care. Health care facilities seek JCAHO accreditation voluntarily. JCAHO defines a standard as "a statement of expectation that defines the structures and processes that must be substantially in place in an organization to enhance the quality of care" (JCAHO, 1995, p. 655). JCAHO has identified standards for measuring the performance of services provided by health care organizations. JCAHO (1995, p. 551) states that an organization is responsible to "ensure that the same level of quality of patient care is provided."

JCAHO requires interdisciplinary coordination of performance improvement (PI) efforts throughout a health care organization. Achieving continuous improvement in care requires collaboration between administrative services (such as medical records, fiscal service) and clinical services (for example, nursing, medicine, pharmacy). JCAHO reviews the extent to which health care organizations (hospitals, nursing homes, outpatient clinics) meet the JCAHO's written PI standards.

American Nurses Association Standards of Clinical Nursing Practice. In keeping abreast of changes in health care, the American Nurses Association (ANA) updated the standards of the profession. The ANA Standards of Clinical Nursing Practice, 1991 (Appendix K) define the nurse's role in the delivery of nursing care to a client or group of clients, which "may be provided in the context of disease or injury prevention, health promotion, health restoration, or health maintenance" (ANA, 1991, p. 1).

The ANA Standards of Clinical Nursing Practice "are authoritative statements by which the nursing profession describes the responsibilities for which its practitioners are accountable" (ANA, 1991, p. 1). The Standards provide clients and nurses with written criteria against which the nurse's actual performance is compared and measured, thus this is a step toward ensuring delivery of consistent, competent nursing care to all clients. The ANA Standards are the basis for measuring performance improvement in the delivery of nursing care.

The ANA Standards of Clinical Nursing Practice are divided into Standards of Care and Standards of Professional Performance. Standards of Care "describe a competent level of nursing care as demonstrated by the nursing process, involving assessment, diagnosis, outcome identification, planning, implementation, and evaluation. The nursing process encompasses all significant actions taken by nurses in providing care to all clients and forms the foundation of clinical decision making" (ANA, 1991, pp. 2–3). Annual performance appraisals (evaluations) of nursing performance reflect the nurses' ability to implement the nursing process. Standards of Professional Performance (ANA, 1991, p. 2) "describe a competent level of behavior in the professional role." The standards embrace the following aspects of behavior:

- the quality of care
- performance appraisal
- education
- collegiality
- ethics
- collaboration
- research
- resource utilization

Clinical Practice Guidelines

Clinical practice guidelines delineate the care, course of action, or tactical plan for specific situations. Guidelines are not policies or recipes. They are recommended practices and may be generated at the national level (for example, prediction and prevention of pressure ulcers in adult clients) or at a local health care facility to meet the specific needs of a client population served (for example, foot care for clients with diabetes). Guidelines describe a process of client care management that has the potential of improving the quality of clinical and consumer decision making.

Agency for Health Care Policy and Research. At the national level, guidelines are established by the Agency for Health Care Policy and Research (AHCPR). The agency is a component of the US Department of Health and Human Services and was created by Congress to control Medicare spending by devising and promoting clinical practice guidelines. The intent of the research-based guidelines was to make positive contributions to the quality of care in the United States by assisting clinicians and clients to make decisions about appropriate health care for specific clinical conditions.

AHCPR generates and disseminates research findings and guidelines to health care providers, policymakers, and the public. "Guidelines are systematically developed statements to assist practitioner and patient decisions about appropriate health care for specific clinical conditions" (AHCPR, 1992, p. ii).

An independent, interdisciplinary panel of experts representing nursing, medicine, pharmacy, nutrition and other disciplines developed the guidelines. The guidelines are specific to clinical conditions (acute pain, urinary incontinence, stroke) and assist nurses and other health team members by describing recommended courses of action for various clinical situations, specific client conditions, or populations. The guidelines provide linkages among diagnoses or clinical conditions, interventions, and outcomes. Practitioners (nurses) arrive at a decision to adopt the guidelines using available resources and adapt them to the circumstances presented by clients (AHCPR, 1995). The guidelines contribute to the quality of care in the United States by striving to identify a course of action that leads to the same level of care for similar problems (urinary incontinence).

Continuum of Care

Health care organizations view the clients' care as part of a continuum that over time enables clients to have access to an integrated system of settings, services, and care levels (JCAHO, 1995). The continuum of care is provided over an extended period of time, in various settings, and spans illness to wellness. Use of the problem-solving approach organizes the thinking processes of clinicians to plan and implement the client's care in an organized manner throughout the continuum of care. Thinking logically reduces the enormity of the problems presented to clinicians daily. The continuum of care involves matching the client's needs with the appropriate level and type of medical, health, or social service. Coordination of care is required in order to guide the client through the health care system and integrate the components of care from the preentry phase through the exit phase. The interdisciplinary team members, especially the discharge planner, coordinate the delivery of care between clinical services in an organization and with community health agencies external to the organization. Current delivery models of health care focus on providing a consistent, outcome driven plan of care. A case management approach assists clinicians in guiding the client through the continuum of care.

Case Management

Case management organizes care to ensure that specific client outcomes are achieved within prescribed time frames through the use of appropriate resources. The care is coordinated by a case manager (nurse, social worker, nurse practitioner) who follows the client through a continuum of care that may include an inpatient stay in the hospital, followed by clinic visits in ambulatory care settings or care delivered in a nursing home, the client's home, or hospice centers. The case manager ensures that the interdisciplinary team members are fulfilling their responsibilities to the clients in achieving identified outcomes. Clinical pathways may be used to guide the delivery of the same level of competent care.

Primary care, a case management approach, evolved when the locus of client care continued to shift from the inpatient setting to the outpatient clinic. Today hospitalized clients are discharged earlier, and many conditions for which clients were traditionally hospitalized are now managed entirely in the ambulatory care setting. Statistics reflect that there has been a decrease in the length of hospital inpatient stays and an increase in the number of outpatient clinic visits. The client is assigned to a primary care team. The primary care team may consist of physicians, nurse practitioners, and registered nurses. The client sees the same practitioners at each clinic visit, and the team assumes responsibility for guiding the client's progress through the continuum of care.

Interdisciplinary Care Plans

The framework for case management involves a collaborative interdisciplinary team approach to care, the development of a comprehensive case management plan, implementation of a clinical pathway to guide care, and concurrent analysis, evaluation, and adjustment of the care rendered. The interdisciplinary clinical experts (nursing, medical, dietary, pharmaceutic, respiratory, physical therapy, social service, utilization review) unite to determine the sequence and timing of interventions and outcomes for particular medical and nursing diagnoses or diagnosis-related groups and, at the same time, promote the appropriate and effective use of resources, human and financial. Facilities may choose to replace the nursing care plan with an interdisciplinary care plan, and the nursing components of care are then incorporated into the interdisciplinary plan. Once the interdisciplinary plans of care (see Appendix L) are implemented, the interdisciplinary team meets regularly (weekly) to review the plans and the attainment of identified outcomes. Reviewing the plan on a regular basis allows the team to ascertain the plan's effectiveness. For example, an interdisciplinary team in psychiatry may consist of psychiatrists, psychologists, psychiatric staff nurses, psychiatric clinical nurse specialist, social worker, dietitian, and recreational therapist, and the team meets to discuss the progress of clients in meeting the outcomes identified on their interdisciplinary plans of care.

Clinical Pathways

Another popular avenue for helping to ensure the delivery of consistent, competent care is the development and implementation of clinical pathways, also called critical pathways or care maps. Clinical pathways are interdisciplinary guidelines for rendering care to specific client populations. Usually the specific diagnoses identified on clinical pathways reflect high-volume, high-risk, and high-cost cases. Health care facilities develop pathways for specific populations such as clients with newly diagnosed diabetes, congestive heart failure, human immunodeficiency virus (HIV), or tuberculosis.

The pathways lead the provider along a sequence of interdisciplinary interventions that incorporate client and family education, discharge plans, consultations, and information about nutrition, medications, activities, diagnostics, therapeutics, and treatments. In addition, clients walk along the path until they reach their destinations, the outcomes. In many organizations, clinical pathways are replacing the traditional nursing care plans and interdisciplinary care plans. Clinical pathways are outcome-driven and provide a time line to achieve the expected outcomes. Health care providers project that pathways will lead to reduced costs of care and shorter inpatient hospital stays. Variances, that is, departures from the expected pathway, may occur as a result of unexpected changes in a client's condition or lack of resources necessary to complete the pathway.

■ MEASURING PERFORMANCE IMPROVEMENT

Change has been effected in the monitoring of care. The health care system has shifted from a quality assurance methodology that focused on meeting thresholds (90% compliance) to continuous performance improvement. Today, health care organizations systematically measure, evaluate, and improve their performance to effect successful client health outcomes (JCAHO, 1995). A measure may be a standard or an indicator, which is a tool to measure an organization's performance over time. For example, an indicator may measure the effect of the nurse's teaching on a newly diagnosed diabetic client's ability to administer the prescribed insulin to himself.

Nursing service, in collaboration with other services, constructs PI activities that quantitatively measure the organization's and nursing's contribution to improving client care. Sharing results of the PI activities assists the organization and nurses in recognizing areas that require improvement. Student nurses and practicing professionals contribute to the PI process to ensure the delivery of consistent, competent client care. For example, a PI monitor may measure the effect of the problem-solving approach on helping the client prepare for continuing care after discharge from the inpatient setting.

Measuring improvements is conducted through the use of benchmarks. Benchmarking was first used by the Xerox Corporation in the late 1970s to improve organizational performance through systematic identification and implementation of best practices. Xerox defined benchmarking as the continuous process of measuring products, services, and practices against companies acclaimed as industry leaders.

In nursing, benchmarking may be used to compare the performance of the nursing staff in achieving successful client outcomes with the staff in other facilities of the same size and similar client population. For example, clients with indwelling catheters in one nursing home may experience fewer urinary tract infections per inpatient days than at another facility. The second nursing home facility in this situation would use benchmarking for problem solving and develop strategies to decrease the number of infections. Comparing the performance of nursing staff internally and with community standards reflects the current trend in health care practice.

■ MALPRACTICE: FAILURE TO IMPLEMENT PROFESSIONAL STANDARDS

Failure to implement professional standards may lead to professional negligence, resulting in malpractice litigation against the nurse, the interdisciplinary team, and the health care organization. Specifically, malpractice stems from incorrect treatment (for example, giving the wrong medication, resulting in harm to a client) or negligent treatment (failure to implement established protocol) of a client by health care team members (physician, dentist, nurse) responsible for health care. For the plaintiff (client or family) to be compensated for damages, the plaintiff establishes the following elements:

- the existence of the nurse's duty to the plaintiff, based on the existence of the nurse–patient relationship
- the applicable standard of nursing care and the nurse's violation of this standard
- a compensable injury, one for which the injured client is entitled to receive payment for damages
- a causal connection between the violation of the standard of care and the harm the client claimed (Black et al, 1990).

Registered nurses are legally bound to follow the ANA Standards of Clinical Nursing Practice. In a malpractice suit against a registered nurse, the plaintiff's attorney will evaluate whether the nurse, who is the defendant in the malpractice suit, implemented professional standards of practice, that is, the nursing standards that a reasonable and prudent nurse would be expected to follow.

The ANA Standards of Clinical Nursing Practice permit nurses to:

- defend their practices if the need arises
- conduct research to improve nursing practice
- measure the actual nursing care provided to clients against an established standard for quality and appropriateness

The Relationship of Critical Thinking, Problem Solving, Nursing Process, and Decision Making

Critical thinking, problem solving, nursing process, and decision making are the crucial, intricately meshed steps that guide patient care.

■ CRITICAL THINKING

Critical thinking is an invisible process, a mental activity that renders visible shape to the data gathered throughout the interdisciplinary team's clinical interactions with clients and families. From the moment a team member (for example, a nurse) sees a client and listens to his or her problems and concerns, the team member develops ideas about the cause and treatment of the problem. The team members learn about the clients as people, the meaning of the illness to the clients and others, and its impact on their lives.

Critical thinking continues as the team members gather the health history and perform physical examinations. Findings from these two sources raise or lower the likelihood of certain problems or diagnoses. The findings may exclude some of the nurse's initial ideas about what is wrong with the clients or open up new avenues for exploration.

In order to perform critical thinking, nurses learn the basic concepts of anatomy, physiology, chemistry, nutrition, microbiology, psychology, and sociology (including culture, spiritual orientation, education) to develop a scientific social base to allow nurses to conduct initial assessments and reassessments of the clients' physiologic, psychologic, social, cultural, and spiritual status. Nurses learn pathology (involving abnormalities in body structures), pathophysiology (physiologic processes altered by disease), and psychopathology (disorders of mood or thinking). The acquired body of knowledge forms the basis for recognizing change during subsequent assessments and reassessments. Critical thinking facilitates the identification of contributing factors, both positive and negative, that determine the clients' location on the health-through-illness continuum. The direction the client is facing on the continuum is more important than actual placement on the continuum. A client may be physically debilitated while maintaining a positive attitude toward life and self-care. This client will be facing toward achieving an optimal state of health, wellness, and well-being.

EXAMPLE OF A HEALTH TO ILLNESS CONTINUUM

Health<<<<<<<<<<<<<<<^>>>>>>>>>>>>>>Illness
Midpoint

The nurses' knowledge base includes an awareness of interpersonal skills (the ability to interact with the clients) to garner the necessary information, the fundamentals of problem-solving analysis exemplified through the nursing process, and competencies in decision making (clinical judgment). Through implementation of the nursing process, nurses analyze the assessment data, recognize significant relationships among the data and cluster similar data, develop valid conclusions (identifying nursing diagnoses) through synthesis of the data, and subsequently, make sound nursing judgments (deciding on plans, outcomes, and interventions) that contribute to the clients' progress.

Critical thinkers support their own viewpoints with facts (evidence), reflect independent thinking, do not rely on others to make judgments for them, possess the good sense to seek assistance as needed, determine priorities of care, and focus on meeting urgent needs first.

Interdisciplinary teams base care decisions on information developed about each client's needs and the response of the client to the therapeutic regimen. Making care decisions reflects critical (orderly) thinking and implementation of the problem-solving approach and the nursing process. The interdisciplinary team employs critical thinking to refine the enormous amount of information gathered, draw conclusions, and make decisions regarding care.

■ PROBLEM SOLVING AND NURSING PROCESS

The problem-solving approach facilitates continuity of care provided over an extended time, in various settings, and spanning the illness-to-wellness continuum. The problem-solving approach is a form of critical thinking and provides a framework for facilitating the identification of solutions that lead to successful client outcomes. The problem-solving approach is not unique to health care and is also used in business and research. For example, Total Quality Improvement activities incorporate the problem-solving approach in identifying areas within an organization that represent opportunities for improvement, for example, the safe administration of medications.

The admission of clients with complex problems for short hospital stays and clients scheduled for outpatient clinic visits compels the registered nurse to quickly and systematically collect information from the client and family, identify problems, and initiate a course of action to resolve each problem. The orderly manner in which the nurse performs the steps is called the problem-solving approach.

The problem-solving approach is a continuous systematic method of assessing human responses to health problems and developing written care plans aimed at resolving the problems. For example, intensive care units, psychiatric units, and nursing home care units develop interdisciplinary plans of care. The health problems identified by the nurse and the interdisciplinary team may be related to the client, family, or the community. The problem-solving approach, incorporated into the nursing process, is reflected in the following phases:

- **PHASE 1:** Assessment and Reassessment
- **PHASE 2:** Diagnosis of Problem or Deficit
- **PHASE 3:** Planning and Outcome Identification
- **PHASE 4:** Implementation
- **PHASE 5:** Evaluation of Outcomes

Nurses strive to resolve health problems through the **problem-solving approach.** The phases are graphically depicted in the problem-solving **cycle** (Figure 2–1). The cycle begins when the client enters the health care delivery system.

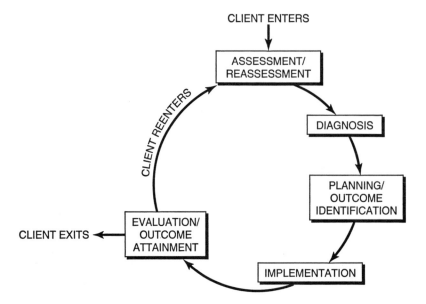

Figure 2–1. Nursing Process and Problem-Solving Cycle

TABLE 2–1. COMPARISON OF PROBLEM-SOLVING APPROACH, NURSING PROCESS, AND SCIENTIFIC METHOD

Problem Solving	Nursing Process	Scientific Method
• Collection of information	• Assessment	• Observe phenomena
• Identify a problem	• Diagnosis	• Identify question
• Specify expected outcomes	• Plan and outcomes	• Hypothesis
• Generation of alternative courses of action		• Establish method
• Activate the plan	• Implementation of plan	• Procedural steps
• Examine the end results	• Evaluation of outcomes	• Measure, analyze, and synthesize the findings
		• Discuss the findings and state conclusions

- The nurse initiates the first phase of the cycle, **assessment,** by gathering data from the client and family and **reassesses** the client throughout the course of treatment.
- A **diagnosis** related to the client's problem or chief complaint is identified in the second phase.
- Within the third phase, the nurse and client work together to formulate a **plan** of action and **identify outcomes** aimed at resolving the client's problem.
- During the fourth phase, the plan is **implemented** by the nurse, the interdisciplinary team, the client, and the family, when appropriate.
- In the fifth phase, the interdisciplinary team, the nurse, and the client **evaluate** whether the outcomes have been achieved and the problem resolved. The client exits the cycle if the outcomes have been achieved.
- The client reenters the cycle if the outcomes were not achieved and the interdisciplinary team reinitiates the first phase in the problem-solving process by reassessing the client.

The problem-solving approach helps to identify human responses to health problems. Human responses represent changes in the client's sense of well-being, wellness, and life-style. Plans and pathways customize the delivery of nursing care to each client, aid in problem resolution, and provide evidence that measurable outcomes were attained.

Consistent implementation of the problem-solving approach is essential throughout a school of nursing and a health care center. Consistency in teaching helps the student and practicing nurse to transfer learning from the classroom to the clinical setting.

The problem-solving approach is similar to the nursing process and the scientific method (Table 2–1). A problem is a question that is put forth for solution. For example, what is the relationship between the fre-

quency of turning comatose clients and the incidence of pressure ulcers? The problem indicated in this question is the incidence of pressure ulcers; one proposed solution is the frequency of turning the client. Another question might be, what is the effect of structured preoperative teaching on the client's ability to effectively manage pain postoperatively? The problem in this situation is postoperative pain management; one solution is structured preoperative teaching.

■ DECISION MAKING

In making decisions, the interdisciplinary team promotes consideration of client values and preferences, including the decision to discontinue treatment. Clients are involved in the following aspects of their care:

- giving informed consent
- making care decisions
- resolving dilemmas about care decisions
- formulating advance directives
- withholding resuscitative services
- forgoing or withdrawing life-sustaining treatment
- care at the end of life

The family may participate in care decisions; however, clients have a right to exclude any or all family members from participating in their care decisions (JCAHO, 1995, p. 84). A surrogate decision maker is someone appointed to act on behalf of another. Surrogates make decisions only when a client is without capacity or has given permission to involve others. Health care organizations have a process for resolving dilemmas about care decision. For example, when a decision by a health care provider (such as a physician) differs from the expressed wishes of the client or surrogate, the matter may be referred to an Ethics Committee for recommendation.

Assessment and Reassessment

The purpose of the initial assessment, or screening, is to gather specific information (data) from the client and family to establish a database in the health care system. Authority to perform assessments and reassessments and formulate diagnoses is derived from several sources:

- state and federal laws
- licensure
- national certification
- national, state, and community standards
- institutional (medical center) standards, policies, procedures, and protocols

The data are compared with other data collected in the delivery of care to measure the effectiveness of prescribed therapeutic regimens. The client's physical, psychologic, cultural, and social status are assessed, analyzed, synthesized, and problems are identified. The *American Nurses Association Standards of Clinical Practice* (1991) states:

Standard I Assessment: The nurse systematically evaluates the quality and effectiveness of nursing practice.

The following flow chart (Figure 3–1) demonstrates the assessment and reassessment phase and focuses on the importance of three activities:

- gathering data initially and throughout the client's contact with the health care facility
- analyzing the data to create information about the client's needs
- decision making to select appropriate care and treatment interventions

Assessments and reassessments are tailored to collect data on specific client populations. For example, the interdisciplinary team at a medical-surgical fa-

cility collects data related to current problems, past history, client's cultural and spiritual orientation, nutritional status, daily activity level, educational level, vocational status, medicine usage, cognition, and communication skills. Nurses in a nursing home, on the other hand, tailor their assessments to identify cognitive and physical deficits that may lead to safety hazards. Of concern are falls, nutritional status, the interaction of the drugs the client receives, interactions of the drugs clients receive with the food they eat, and the level of capacity for independent activity.

Clients' needs are assessed and reassessed by nurses employed at various community health care agencies. Hospice center nurses focus on improving the client's quality of life until death and assess the management of pain. The staffs of rehabilitation centers assess the client's function in physical, mental, social, economic, and vocational areas of their lives. Nurses assess clients in physicians' offices. Nurses working at ambulatory care centers located in urban and rural settings assess the clients at scheduled clinic visits and at unplanned visits to an emergency room. Industrial nurses focus on assessing employees' health status and advocating healthy life-styles. The interdisciplinary team members at crisis centers may provide 24-hour telephone service to help people cope with an immediate crisis, and provide subsequent support for long-term care. Home health care agency nurses assess the clients in their homes and provide interventions that maximize independent functioning of the client. Nurses employed by state, county, or city public health agencies assess the needs of the community and offer programs to meet the health needs of the people.

Another client population for whom specific data are tailored includes persons who are chemically dependent. The data collected from clients seeking treatment for alcoholism or other drug dependencies in-

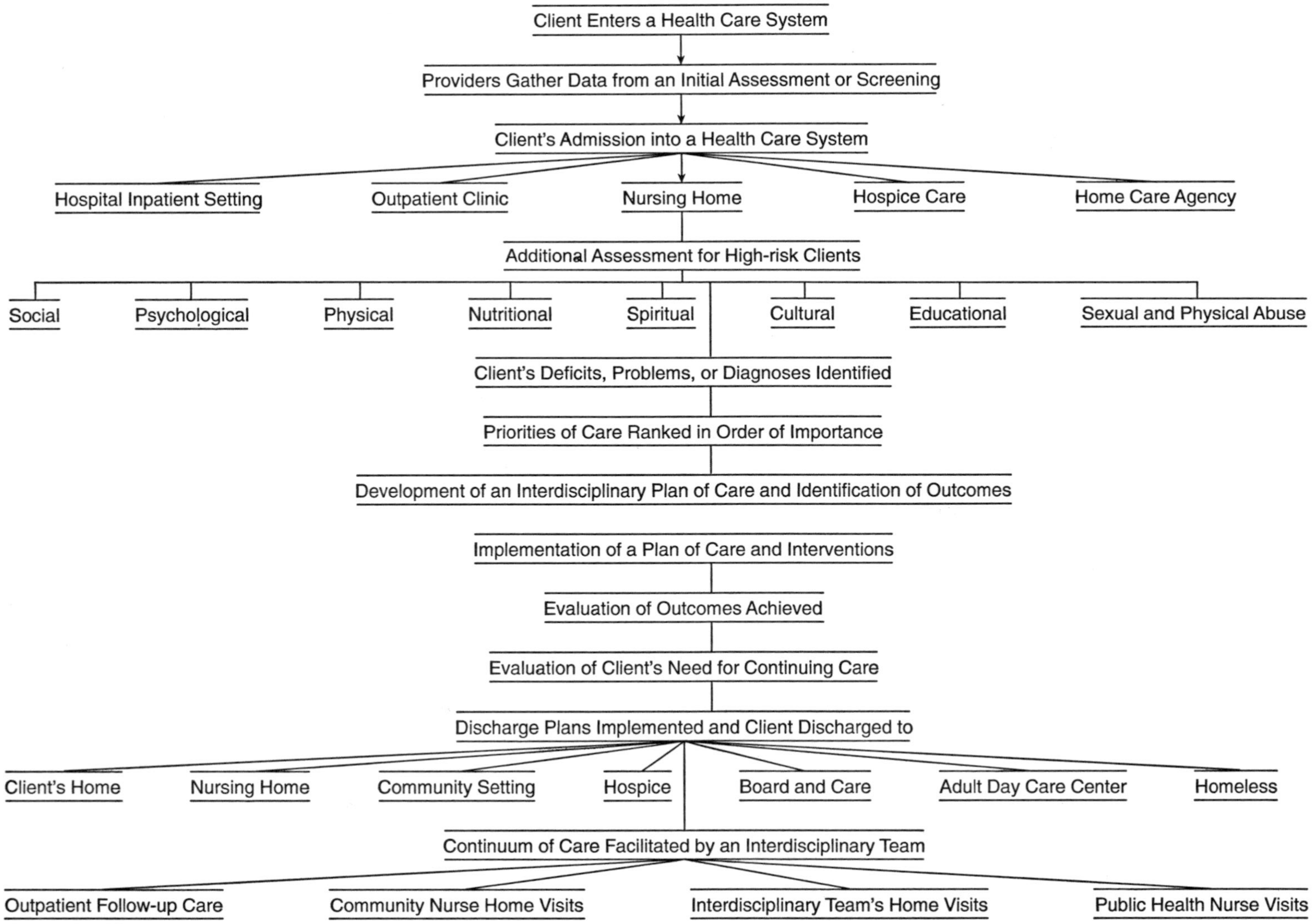

Figure 3–1. Continuum of Care

clude history of alcohol and illicit drug use; history of physical problems; alcohol and illicit drug use by family members; the spiritual orientation of the patient; the types of previous treatment and responses to the treatment; history of physical or sexual abuse.

Nurses assessing pediatric clients determine developmental age; length; height; weight; head circumference; immunization record; nutritional status; and emotional, cognitive, educational, social, and daily activity needs.

■ JCAHO STANDARD ON ASSESSMENT

JCAHO standards specify that "an assessment with at least a history, physical examination, and nursing care assessment are completed within 24 hours of admission. The time frame applies for weekday, weekend, and holiday admissions" (JCAHO, 1995, p. 111). JCAHO standards also state that "a registered nurse assesses the patient's need for nursing care in all settings in which nursing care is to be provided" (JCAHO, 1995, p. 105). For example, if a client is receiving home care, a registered nurse will conduct the initial assessment and subsequently identify and establish the priorities of care in collaboration with the client and family.

In accordance with organization policy, registered nurses determine the priorities of a client's care at the time of an initial assessment and in collaboration with other interdisciplinary team members. Through the years, Maslow's hierarchy of needs (p. 16) has been successfully used by various health care disciplines in identifying high-, medium-, and low-priority needs. Other qualified nursing staff members (licensed practical nurses or licensed vocational nurses, mental health technicians, or nursing assistants) can assist the registered nurses with the assessment process. Delegated aspects of the assessment process are carried out in accordance with applicable laws and regulations and established hospital policies and procedures (JCAHO, 1995).

■ INTERDISCIPLINARY ASSESSMENT

The shift toward interdisciplinary collaboration creates a need to develop a framework for practice that is amenable to all disciplines. The trend is toward an interdisciplinary assessment of the client. Then, priority problems are identified, diagnoses agreed upon, an interdisciplinary plan of care and outcomes formulated, the plan executed, and the outcomes evaluated.

When clients enter the health care system, qualified providers assess the clients' need for care throughout their contact with the facility. To help ensure consistency in assessment, staff at the health care facility define in writing the scope (range) of the assessments performed by each clinical discipline. These definitions are integrated into policies and procedures, protocols, or other documented guidelines. The policies conform with state licensure laws, applicable regulations, and certification.

The requirements for assessment may differ for each health care facility; therefore, providers (registered nurses) review the policies at each health care facility before delivering care. Student nurses also review the policies of affiliating health care facilities before beginning their clinical experience. Following are policies that documents define:

- the data gathered to assess client needs
- the scope of assessment by each discipline (nursing, medicine, physical therapy)
- the mechanisms designed to analyze the data to determine the approach to meet clients' needs
- the framework for decision making based on the analysis of the information

For example, while conducting admission physical examinations, providers (registered nurse, physician, dietitian) inspect clients for manifestations of nutrient deficiency or excess and the effect of medications on nutritional status. Providers may explore the effect of the clients' religious, cultural, ethical beliefs and personal food preferences on their daily nutritional intake. A health care organization's policy on assessment may indicate that a dietetian will assess clients at high risk for nutritional deficits. The nutritional assessment may include the client's medical, nutritional, and medication histories; physical examination; food allergies; anthropometric measurements; height and weight; skin fold evaluation for subcutaneous fat examination; and laboratory data (serum albumin level, hemoglobin).

■ CONFIDENTIALITY OF INFORMATION

Information (data) obtained from the client, family, and other sources is kept secure and confidential by nurses and other health team members. Information is restricted to individuals who have a need for it and who have permission for access. Access to the clients' computerized medical records is controlled by information management services.

■ INTEGRATING MODELS

To facilitate the gathering and analysis of data, a model (design) may serve as a framework for organizing and clarifying information and showing the interrelationships among the data collected. Various types of frameworks are used in nursing practice: nonnursing models, such as body systems; and nursing models, such as nursing theories and Gordon's Functional Health Patterns. In practice, a nurse may combine models, for example, a body systems approach and a functional health pattern.

Nonnursing Assessment Models

Examples of nonnursing models are:

- a head-to-toe assessment: a cephalocaudal approach
- the body systems method, called a medical model
- Maslow's Hierarchy of Needs

A head-to-toe assessment begins with the nurse inspecting and examining the client's body, beginning at the client's head and progressing down to the toes (Fig. 3–2).

Assessment of clients by body systems (Table 3-1), a medical model, has been the dominant assessment framework used in health care and the one traditionally employed by physicians. Data collection includes both historical (subjective) and physical (objective) cues, and findings are reported within the context of a disease or medical diagnosis. This assessment framework has been used effectively by physicians and clearly reflects phenomena of concern to the discipline. Over the years this medical model served as a guide to data collection for other health care providers, including nurses. In a medical model, a medical diagnosis (myocardial infarction) addresses pathologic cellular, tissue, and organ changes. Changes are identified through an assessment of body systems, for example, the cardiovascular system.

Maslow's Hierarchy of Needs (Fig. 3–3), a nonnursing model, contends that all people have the same basic human needs. The physiologic needs are met first, and then the individual progresses through the higher levels of safety and security, love and belonging, self-esteem, and self-actualization.

Nursing Assessment Models

Nursing assessment models deal with human responses to problems that nurses can treat. A nursing model may be adapted to incorporate the requirements of other disciplines and may serve as the framework for data collection of data by other disciplines (such as dietetics). Assessment models developed by nursing theorists offer an alternative assessment perspective. Data collection is guided by the framework of the theory. Examples of nursing theories employed in nursing curricula and clinical practice are Hender-

son's Nature of Nursing (1966); Orem's Self-Care Theory (Orem, 1971); and Roy's Adaptation Model (1976).

Functional Health Patterns is a typology that links assessment and human responses to actual or potential health problems (Gordon, 1994). The framework focuses the attention of nurses on the behaviors manifested by clients within each of 11 functional health patterns. The data collected are evaluated against parameters (limits) that reflect expected responses for a given age group, stage of development, culture, health status, and personal values and beliefs. The framework focuses on content that is within the scope of nursing and leads to the identification of nursing diagnoses, interventions, and outcomes for which the nurse is clearly accountable.

Gordon's 11 Functional Health Patterns. (See Chapter 8 for additional information)

1. **Health Perception-Health Management Pattern:** The client's perceived pattern of health and well-being
2. **Nutritional-Metabolic Pattern:** The client's nutritional intake; fluid and electrolyte balance; and condition of skin, hair and nails, height and weight
3. **Elimination Pattern:** The client's patterns of excretory function of the bowel, bladder, and skin
4. **Activity-Exercise Pattern:** The client's pattern of exercise and activity and respiratory and circulatory functions
5. **Sleep-Rest Pattern:** The client's patterns of sleep, rest, and perception of energy level
6. **Cognitive-Perceptual Pattern:** The client's patterns of hearing, vision, taste, touch, smell, pain perception, language, memory and decision making
7. **Self-Perception and Self-Concept Pattern:** The client's attitudes about self and perception of abilities
8. **Role-Relationships Pattern:** The client's role and relationships with family
9. **Sexuality-Reproductive Pattern:** The client's actual perceived satisfaction or problems with sexuality
10. **Coping-Stress Tolerance Pattern:** The clients' ability to manage stress and the use of support systems
11. **Value-Belief Pattern:** The client's patterns of values, beliefs including spiritual ones, or goals that guide choices or decisions

CHIEF COMPLAINT
Client's description of the present problem

DEMOGRAPHIC DATA
Age, race, sex, place of birth, marital status, occupation, residence, telephone number, health insurance, dominant language, highest educational level, and cultural, religious, and spritual beliefs.
Source of the history
Reliability of the source (1–4)

GENERAL APPEARANCE
Well-groomed; disheveled; soiled clothes; oriented to time, place, person, and situation
Color: pink, pale, red, jaundiced, mottled, blanched, cyanotic
Skin: rashes, lesions, lumps, dryness, color changes in hair or nails, presence of lice or scabies, temperature, turgor

PAST HISTORY
State of health from the client's point of view
Childhood illnesses
Adult illnesses
Psychiatric illness
Accidents and injuries
Surgery
Emergency room visits
Current health promotion practices
Current medications
Environmental allergies

Use of tobacco, alcohol, drugs, caffeine
Diet; typical daily intake of food and fluids
Screening tests
Immunizations
Sleep patterns
Planned exercise
Environmental hazards at work; use of safety devices

FAMILY HISTORY
Age, health, or cause of death of each immediate family member
History of disease present in the family
History of psychological problems in the family
Home situation and relationship with others
Typical day in the life of the client

VITAL SIGNS
Temperature
Pulse: apical, radial
Respirations
Blood pressure: supine, sitting, standing; right and left arms
Height and weight compared with average for frame

HEAD AND FACE
Size, contour, symmetry, color, pain, tenderness, lesions, edema
Scalp: color, texture, scales, lumps, lesions, inflammation, infestation
Face: movement, expression, pigmentation, acne, tics, tremors, scars

EYES
Acuity: visual loss, glasses, contacts, prosthesis, double vision, blurred vision, photophobia, color vision, pain, burning, excessive tearing
Eyelid: color, ptosis, edema, styes, exophthalmos
Extraocular movement: position and alignment of eyes, strabismus, nystagmus
Conjunctiva: color, discharge, vascular changes
Iris: color, markings
Sclera: color, vascularity, jaundice
Pupils: size, shape, equality, reaction to light

EARS
Acuity: hearing loss, use of hearing aid, earache, dizziness, ringing in the ear, sensitivity to sound
External ear: lobe, auricle, canal
Inner ear: vertigo

NOSE
Smell, nasal size, symmetry, flaring, sneezing, deformities
Mucosa: color, edema, exudate, bleeding, furuncle, pain, tenderness, nosebleeds
Sinus: tenderness, pain

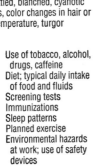

MOUTH AND THROAT
Odor, pain, ability to speak, bite, chew, swallow, taste
Lips: color, symmetry, hydration, lesions, crusting, fever blisters, cracking, swelling, numbness, drooling
Gums: color, edema, bleeding, retraction, pain
Teeth: number, missing, caries, caps, dentures, sensitivity to heat or cold
Tongue: symmetry, color, size, hydration, markings, protrusion, ulcers, burning, swelling, coating
Throat: gag reflex, soreness, cough, sputum, hemoptysis
Voice: hoarseness, loss, change in pitch

NECK
Symmetry, movement, range of motion, masses, scars, pain or stiffness, swollen glands
Trachea: deviation, scars
Thyroid: size, shape, symmetry, tenderness, enlargement, nodules, scars
Vessels: quality, strength and symmetry of pulsations, bruits, venous distention
Lymph nodes: size, shape, mobility, tenderness, enlargement

CHEST
Size, shape, symmetry, deformities, pain, tenderness
Skin: color, rashes, scars, hair distribution, turgor, temperature, edema, crepitation
Breast: contour, symmetry, color, size, shape, inflammation, scars, masses, pain, dimpling, swelling
Nipples: color, discharge ulceration, bleeding, inversion, pain
Axillae: nodes, enlargement, tenderness, rash, inflammation

LUNGS
Breathing patterns: rate, regularity, depth, ease, normal, fremitus, use of accessory muscles
Sounds: normal, adventitious (crackling, wheezing, gurgling, rubbing), intensity, pitch, quality, duration, equality, vocal resonance

HEART
Cardiac patterns: rate, rhythm, slow heartbeat, rapid heartbeat, intensity, regularity, skipped or extra beats, chest pain, implanted pacemaker

BACK
Scars, sacral edema, spinal abnormalities, kyphosis, scoliosis, tenderness, pain

KIDNEY
Urinary output, frequency, urgency, hesitancy, burning, pain, dribbling, incontinence, hematuria, nocturia, oliguria

GENITALIA
Female
Labia majora and minora
Urethral and vaginal orifices: discharge, swelling, ulceration, nodules, masses, tenderness, pain
Male
Penis: discharge, ulceration, pain
Scrotum: color, size, nodules, swelling, ulcerations, tenderness
Testes: size, shape, swelling, masses, absence

RECTUM
Pigmentation, hemorrhoids, excoriation, rashes, abscess, pilonidal cyst, masses, lesions, tenderness, pain, itching, burning

EXTREMITIES
Size, shape, symmetry, range of motion, temperature, color, pigmentation, scars, hematomas, bruises, rash, ulceration, numbness, paresis, swelling, gait and balance, prosthesis, fracture
Joints: symmetry, active and passive mobility, deformities, stiffness, fixation, masses, swelling fluid, crepitation, pain, tenderness
Muscles: symmetry, size, shape, tone, weakness, cramps, spasms, rigidity, tremor
Vessels: symmetry and strength of pulses, venous filling, varicosities, phlebitis

NEUROLOGIC
Involuntary movements, weakness, paralysis, seizures, numbness or loss of sensation, tingling

PSYCHIATRIC
Nervousness, tension, paranoia, anorexia, bulimia, depression, memory

Figure 3–2: Head-to-Toe Assessment

TABLE 3–1. ASSESSMENT USING A BODY SYSTEMS APPROACH

1. Integumentary (skin, hair, nails)
2. Respiratory (nose, pharynx, larynx, trachea, bronchi, and lungs)
3. Cardiovascular (heart, blood vessels)
4. Nervous (brain, cranial nerves, spinal cord, spinal nerves, autonomic ganglia, ganglionated trunks and nerves)
5. Muscluoskeletal (muscle and skeleton)
6. Gastrointestinal (stomach and intestines)
7. Genitourinary (genital and urinary organs)
8. Reproductive (reproductive organs)
9. Endocrine (thyroid, pancreas)
10. Psychiatric and Psychological
11. Current health promotion practices (yearly physical examination; use of folk remedies)
12. Home situation and relationship with others (client's perception of self and role in family; influence of social, cultural and spiritual values on life style; community involvement and impact of community values on life style)

NB Traditional medical model modified by author.

■ PHASE ONE: ASSESSMENT/ REASSESSMENT

> ### ■ COMPONENTS OF THE ASSESSMENT STEP
>
> 1. Data collection
> 2. Data validation
> 3. Organizing, grouping, clustering of the data
> 4. Reassessment to collect additional data
> 5. Reporting and recording the data

■ DATA COLLECTION

What information does the nurse and the interdisciplinary team need to know? Data are uninterpreted material, facts, and clinical observations collected during an assessment activity. Data about the client are collected systematically from various sources by means of interview (history taking), observation, and physical examination. For example, the client, family members, community agencies, and medical records provide information on the health status of the client.

The client, however, is the primary source of information, the original provider of data. Secondary sources of information are individuals other than the client or data that already exist. Secondary sources include the client's health record; reports of laboratory and diagnostic tests; family, community, and health team members.

The information is used to establish a database (baseline) for the client. After the initial assessment, the baseline data are reassessed throughout the continuum of care to measure the client's progress toward resolution of the identified problem. The client's baseline values and changes in values thereafter are compared at various times during treatment to established standards.

Designated parts of the assessment and reassessment forms may require completion within 24 hours by a nurse and a physician. Subsequent assessment of high risk clients may take place within 48 to 72 hours. For example, when assessing a diabetic client, the nurse may find that further analysis of the dietary regimen is required. In that case, the nurse initiates a refer-

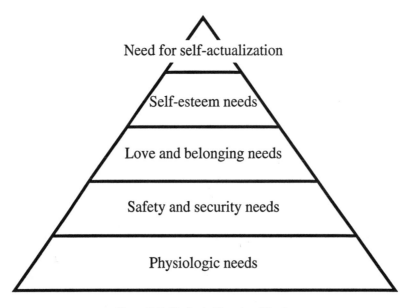

Figure 3–3. Maslow's Hierarchy of Needs

Need for self-actualization

Self-esteem needs

Love and belonging needs

Safety and security needs

Physiologic needs

ral to a dietitian, and the dietitian conducts an in-depth nutritional assessment. Other referrals may be to a chaplain, who may visit a client and assess spiritual needs, or to a physical therapist, who may assess the client for rehabilitation needs.

Possible victims of physical, sexual, or verbal abuse are identified using criteria developed by the health care organization. A provider conducting an initial assessment examines the client's body for bruises and listens to the client's and family's explanations to see if the physical evidence and explanation are compatible. In suspected abuse cases, the provider refers the client to appropriate resources as directed in the health care facility's policy and according to state laws and regulations.

Interdisciplinary assessment and reassessment forms designate which parts are specific to the various disciplines involved in the delivery of care. Numerous discipline-specific assessments may be performed for each client. The data gathered are analyzed. The subsequent integration of information facilitates identifying client needs and establishing priorities. A coordinated, collaborative approach is implemented by the various disciplines. Assessment and reassessment forms may be computer-generated. Computers facilitate the rapid retrieval of data at the point of care.

It is essential to assess the client's individual response to a problem and avoid generalizations about specific cultures or age-specific groups. Human beings respond differently to problems. For example, the different cultural values, beliefs, and religious practices of clients may influence their response to a problem.

Primary Sources for Data Collection
Interview
A method of data collection in which the practitioner (the nurse or physician) interviews the client and family members to obtain responses in a face-to-face encounter. The practitioner gathers information related to the client's past medical history and current complaint.

Physical Examination
The process of inspecting the body and its systems. In performing a physical examination of the client's body, the four procedures are inspection, palpation, percussion, and auscultation.

Inspection (observation) is examination by the eye. The examiner inspects the external surface of the client's body, its movements, and posture. The examiner looks at the client for outward signs. For example, cyanosis, pallor, edema, bleeding, or dilated pupils can be seen by the practitioner. The nurse may observe the movement of the leg to determine if it is in correct alignment. Visual inspections of internal body areas may be conducted using a laryngoscope, broncho-scope, gastroscope, cystoscope, sigmoidoscope, or endoscope.

Auscultation is the process of listening for sounds within the body, usually to sounds of thoracic or abdominal viscera, in order to detect some abnormal condition or to detect fetal heart sounds. A stethoscope is used to amplify sounds. For example, the practitioner assesses the lungs and listens for normal or adventitious breath sounds at each point on the chest. Adventitious breath sounds (crackling, gurgling, or rubbing) are abnormal.

Palpation is the process of applying the hands or fingers to the external surface of the body to detect evidence of disease or abnormalities in the various organs. Palpation is used to determine (1) the texture (hair), (2) temperature (skin), (3) vibration (joint), (4) the position, size, consistency, and mobility of organs or masses, (5) distention (urinary bladder), or (6) presence and rate of peripheral pulses. For example, an empty bladder is not palpable; however, when distended, it is palpable as a smooth and round mass.

Percussion is the use of the examiner's fingers to tap the body lightly but sharply to determine position, size, and consistency of an underlying structure and the presence of fluid or pus in a cavity. These conditions are established by alterations felt and heard in resonance and pitch of the sound emitted, vibration elicited, or resistance encountered. For example, bladder distention may be determined by suprapubic dullness over the bladder.

Secondary Sources for Data Collection
Laboratory
Urinalysis, stool specimens, blood tests and cultures, sputum specimens, or spinal fluid. A urinalysis examines the specimen for color, clarity, odor, sterility, pH, specific gravity, glucose, ketone bodies, and blood. The culture and sensitivity test determine the presence of microorganisms, the type of organism(s), and the antibiotics to which the organism(s) are sensitive.

Other Diagnostic Tests
Roentgenogram (x-ray), electrocardiogram (ECG), computed axial tomograph (CT scan), radioisotope studies, fluoroscopy, sonogram, echogram, and biopsy

SUBJECTIVE DATA

Subjective data, which refer to the client's perceptions and sensations about a health problem, are recorded in the client's history. Subjective data are pieces of information the client describes to the nurse during the nursing assessment interview, such as personal perceptions or feelings of self-worth or pain. Subjective data or symptoms are physical or psychologic feelings that the client experiences and may be a departure from the client's normal sensations (Bates, 1995,). Nurses use quotation marks to record the client's statements in the history and avoid paraphrasing or interpreting the client's responses.

Examples of Subjective Data

"My head is throbbing."	"I hurt all over."
"I feel short of breath."	"My legs feel weak."
"My stomach is burning."	"I feel nervous."
"I am not sleeping at night."	"I feel sad."

Headache, nausea, burning, fatigue, stiffness, shortness of breath, warmth, dizziness, and sadness are sensations the client feels. They are not necessarily visible to the nurse.

 Mr. Lopez Scenario

On 9/8/97, Mr. Lopez arrived at an outpatient clinic for his scheduled appointment, accompanied by his wife Eva. The primary care nurse reviewed Mr. Lopez's medical record, which revealed that Mr. Lopez had yearly physical and dental examinations for the past 10 years. He received immunizations for influenza and a pneumococcal vaccine 2 years ago. Mr. Lopez, aged 67 years, immigrated from Mexico 50 years ago and lives in the southwestern United States. He has been married to Eva for 42 years and they have five children ranging in age from 20 to 40 years old. The 20-year-old son lives at home with his parents while attending a local community college. The other children are married and live in the same neighborhood as their parents. Mr. Lopez's primary language is Spanish, which he speaks at home with the family. He understands, writes, and speaks English. He owns a restaurant specializing in Mexican food and speaks English and Spanish to his employees. The four oldest children work at the restaurant.

After completing the review of the medical record, the nurse initiated an assessment. Mr. Lopez told the nurse, "For the past 2 weeks, I have had to go to the bathroom a lot, and I only pass a little urine." The nurse asked, "Mr. Lopez do you feel a sense of urgency, that is, an immediate need to pass your water?" "Yes, I feel a need to hurry to the bathroom. It burns when I pass my water. It smells strong and is dark orange." The nurse inquired, "How much fluid, that is, water, coffee, or other liquids do you drink each day?" Mr. Lopez responded, "I drink three cups of coffee a day and a tall glass of water at night. My skin feels dry and I have never had that problem before now." The nurse inquired, "What happens when you stand up? Do you feel steady on your feet?" Mr. Lopez said, "Lately, I get dizzy when I stand up." The nurse inquired, "Do you have any pain?" Mr. Lopez explained, "My lower back hurts."

The nurse asked his wife, "Do you have an opportunity to remind your husband to drink more water during the day?" The wife responded, "No hablo ingles. Solamente hablo español." The nurse did not speak Spanish. If the husband had not been present to interpret, the nurse knew the outpatient clinic maintained a list of employees who spoke various languages. Mr. Lopez stated, "My wife only speaks Spanish. She is a good woman and raised our five children while I got our restaurant started. We are a very close family, and every Sunday, we attend the Catholic church in our neighborhood."

The nurse observed that the client was in no acute distress. Vital signs revealed an oral temperature of 38° C (100.4° F), pulse 90, a lying blood pressure of 130/80, and a standing blood pressure of 110/70. Height was 5 feet 7 inches; weight 160 pounds. A urine specimen for urinalysis and a urine specimen for culture and sensitivity were ordered by the physician. The nurse observed that Mr. Lopez's urine specimen was foul-smelling, dark amber, cloudy, and thick. In testing Mr. Lopez's skin turgor, the nurse observed that the skin remained tented and the shape returned in 10 seconds. His fluid intake over a 24-hour period was 780 mL (one cup = 180 mL; one tall glass = 200 mL). The urinalysis revealed a specific gravity (sp gr) >1.030, and the culture and sensitivity report disclosed the presence of *Escherichia coli* with a sensitivity to ampicillin.

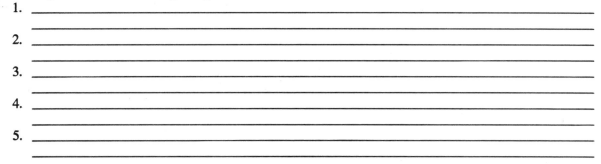

EXERCISE 3–A: *IDENTIFICATION OF SUBJECTIVE DATA*

List the subjective data that Mr. Lopez expressed.

1. _____

2. _____

3. _____

4. _____

5. _____

Correct responses are on p. 29.

OBJECTIVE DATA

Objective data are observed or measured phenomena gathered by someone (registered nurse, physician, nurse practitioner) other than the client and presented factually. For example, the nurse can see the client's respirations and count the rate per minute. In addition, the blood pressure (systolic and diastolic pressure in the arteries) is measured by the practitioner; a numerical reading (130/80) is based on the sounds heard or read on the electronic blood pressure machine. Objective data from primary sources are information collected through the nurses' senses. The nurse can see by observation or inspection (cyanosis of the skin); feel by palpation or percussion (a lump in breast); hear by auscultation or percussion (bowel sounds); or smell (a sweet fruity odor of the breath). Objective data are called signs and reflect the physical and mental manifestations that the practitioner discovers by physical examination and subsequently describes in the client's record as findings (Bates et al, 1995).

Reference laboratory values can provide guidelines for the practitioner when assessing clients by comparison of the subjective and objective data presented by the client with laboratory values. There is no sharp dividing line between normal and abnormal laboratory values. Trends in laboratory values are more valuable than a single value, that is, measuring a value over a period of time. For example, a client with a cholesterol level of 275 mg/dL (reference value <200 mg/dL) may be placed on a low cholesterol diet, and the client's cholesterol level then measured over a 12-month period to determine if the change in diet lowered the level.

Examples of Objective Data
- **Primary source, the client**
  Crackling sounds in the right lower lobe (RLL)
  Stage III pressure ulcer on skin over the coccyx
  Nasal flaring
  Grimacing
  Temperature 100.2° F.
  Respirations 30, shallow
  Cough productive of rusty-brown, purulent sputum

- **Secondary source, the medical record**
  Tuberculin test negative
  Influenza vaccine yearly
  Multiple lobar consolidation on the chest film
  Elevated white blood cell count (WBC) >10,000 mm^3
  Sputum specimen positive for pneumococcal pneumonia

EXERCISE 3–B: *IDENTIFICATION OF OBJECTIVE DATA*

List the objective data demonstrated by Mr. Lopez.

1. _____
2. _____
3. _____
4. _____
5. _____
6. _____
7. _____
8. _____
9. _____

Correct responses are on p. 29.

■ DATA VALIDATION

Do the client's data reflect normal or abnormal findings and standards? Do the objective data support the subjective data? Were data collected accurately?

Whether data reflect a normal measure or range of values is validated by comparing the data with established standards and norms. A standard or norm is an accepted rule or measure. For example, a normal serum electrolyte value for potassium (K^+) is 3.5 to 5.5 mEq/L; a normal hemoglobin (Hgb) for a normal adult man is 14 to 16 g/dL, and for a normal adult woman 12 to 24 g/dL.

The nurse also compares a client's subjective and objective data, verifying that the objective data support the subjective data. For example, if the client states, "I am tired all the time, and cannot play tennis anymore," the nurse may find that the client's Hgb level is below normal for the client's sex and age. The nurse determines whether the client's laboratory results fall within the range of accepted standards and norms. Measurable standards and norms may pertain to vital signs, laboratory findings, diagnostic tests, basic food groups, and growth and development. Reference material should be used by the nurse to document standards and norms.

Documentation may be done in a reference library for the health care staff, or normal ranges for laboratory tests may be found on the printout of the client's laboratory report.

In the following example, the client's test results do not fall within the range of accepted norms.

Comparing Data for Validation

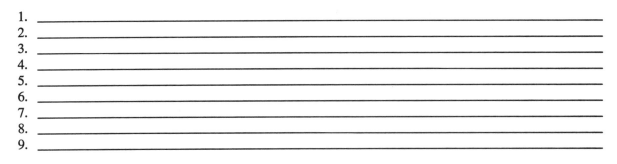

Subjective Data	Objective Date	Standard/ Norm
"My legs feel weak."	Serum K^+ 2.5m EqL	Serum K^+ 3.0–5.5 mEqL
"My blood pressure is usually 110/70."	Blood pressure 170/90 mm Hg	Blood pressure 120/80 mm Hg
"I feel tired all the time."	Hgb 9.0 g/dL	Healthy Adult Female Hgb 12–14 g/dL Male Hgb 14–16g/dL

EXERCISE 3–C: *DATA VALIDATION*

The purpose of exercise 3–C is to learn to compare gathered data with accepted standards and norms to determine the client's abnormal values. Below list subjective data and supporting objective data gathered concerning Mr. Lopez. Compare the client's subjective and objective data with the accepted standards and norms. A list of accepted standards and norms necessary to complete exercise 3–C are located in Appendices F, G, H.

1. Client data

Subjective _____

Objective _____

Normal value _____

2. Client data

Subjective _____

Objective _____

Normal value _____

3. Client data

Subjective _____

Objective _____

Normal value _____

4. Client data

Subjective _____

Objective _____

Normal value _____

5. Client data

Subjective _____

Objective _____

Normal value _____

Correct responses are on p. 29.

■ ORGANIZING (GROUPING, CLUSTERING) DATA

What data are related? After the data are collected, the nurse and health care team members sort through the data and cluster (organize, group) the data to portray a picture of the client's strengths and problems. A cluster forms a composite of similar pieces of data and represents a sequence of behavior over time rather than isolated incidents. Frameworks such as Maslow's Hierarchy of Needs, the 11 Functional Health Patterns, and the use of a body systems approach all aid in the organization of data.

For example, Gordon's 11 Functional Health Patterns help to organize the nursing history and physical examination and to group diagnoses or problem statements. The patterns help the nurse identify the appropriate nursing diagnosis based on the data collected during the initial assessment. All patterns are initially assessed. The data listed under the patterns are analyzed and client problems identified.

With the increased use of preprinted assessment and reassessment forms, data are frequently organized by the structure of the assessment form. For example, data related to nutrition may be grouped together in one section of the assessment form.

Based on the assessment framework selected by a health care facility, clustered data may be grouped under body systems, functional health patterns, or other frameworks. A framework organizes the data collections process and ensures that all pertinent data have been gathered. Information gaps are filled by reassessing the client.

A body system or pattern is deemed functional if the majority of data fall within the range of normal values and standards and represent the client's strengths. A body system or pattern is judged dysfunctional by the nurse if the clustered data fail to meet normal or standard values and represent the client's weaknesses. A dysfunctional body system or pattern may or may not lead to disease. Once the data are clustered, the nurse and other health team members begin to make initial impressions as to the problem.

The following example illustrates clustering of data under a functional health pattern. Accepted standards and norms reveal that the data are not within normal limits; therefore, the pattern is dysfunctional.

Nutritional-Metabolic Pattern
(Gordon's patterns listed on page 14)

Subjective Data	Objective Data	Norm
"I feel nauseated."	Vomited 100 mL	No vomiting
"My skin feels dry."	Skin turgor: skin remained tented 10 seconds	Skin shape returns immediately
"I am thirsty."	24-hour Intake 1000 mL Output 2000 mL	24-hour Intake 2500 mL Output 2500 mL

Body systems approach to the clustering of data

Physicians or other practitioners focus their assessments on a history provided by the client and on examination of the client's body. The medical model does not necessarily assess the cultural, spiritual, and psychosocial needs of the client. The following example illustrates the clustering of data using a body systems approach (see Chapter 9 for additional examples).

General survey: Appears stated age. Sex. Race. Responds appropriately. Clean; neatly groomed. Moves without difficulty. No signs of distress, such as grimacing, labored breathing, continual shifting of feet.

Skin: Normal skin color defined by client's race. Uniformity of color over body. Moist. Skin warm, relatively uniform over the body. Skin turgor: skin returns immediately to normal shape after being lifted, pinched, and released. Skin smooth, soft; moves freely over underlying structures. No lesions. No edema. No odor. Intact.

Hair: Evenly distributed; texture varies from fine to coarse. No infestations. No flaking scalp.

Nails: Smooth; no clubbing or ridges. Nail bed color (normal varies from pink to black pigmentation depending on race). No cyanosis or pallor. Intact tissue surrounding nail beds. Nails well groomed.

Head, Eyes, Ear, Nose, and Throat: **Head:** Symmetrical; scalp smooth; No lesions; facial features symmetrical at rest and with movement. Temporomandibular joint (TMJ) fully movable without pain or crepitation; TMJ opening 3 to 6 cm.

Eyes: Pupils equal, round, reactive to light and accommodation (PERRLA); Extraocular movements (EOMs) intact. Conjunctiva clear; sclera white.

Ears: Hears whispered word at 2 feet (60 cm) bilaterally. Auricles intact bilaterally; canals clear; tympanic membranes intact and without scarring.

Nose: Symmetrical, patent bilaterally; mucous membranes moist, intact with no discharge. Identifies odors accurately.

Mouth/throat: Mucous membrane pink or brown pigmentation in blacks, moist and intact; 32 adult teeth. Uvula midline; active gag reflex. No lesions, areas of irritation, or erosion noted in oral cavity.

Neck: Trachea midline; no palpable nodes. Thyroid not palpable; full range of motion. Carotid pulse is strong, regular bilaterally, and without bruits. No jugular venous distention. Equal strength sternocleidomastoid and trapezius muscles; not taut.

Pulmonary: Anteroposterior (AP) diameter thorax 1:2. Expansion full and equal bilaterally. Lungs clear to percussion and auscultation. Respirations regular rhythm.

Breast: Rounded shape; small, medium, or large nipple. Symmetrical. Skin smooth, intact. Nipple everted, no discharge or lesions. No swelling in axillae. No tenderness, masses, or nodules.

Cardiovascular: Point of maximal impulse (PMI) palpable at fifth intercostal space in midclavicular line. Apical pulse regular rhythm. No extra heart sound; no murmurs noted.

Peripheral Vascular: No edema lower extremities. Extremities warm to touch. Blanch test: nail bed capillaries blanched when pressed and color quickly returned when pressure released.

PERIPHERAL PULSE SCALE
0—Absent
1—Markedly diminished
2—Moderately diminished
3—Slightly diminished
4—Normal

Abdomen: Symmetrical. Positive bowel sounds all quadrants. No masses, no tenderness on palpation. No bruits. Soft, nondistended.

Musculoskeletal: Equal strength bilaterally. Firm hand grasp. Full-range-of-motion in hands, wrists, elbows, shoulders, spine, hips, knees, and ankles. No crepitation or swelling. Even gait; balanced. No joint pain or tenderness. No abnormal curvature of spine.

GRADING MUSCLE STRENGTH

Scale	% Normal Strength	Characteristics
0	0	Complete paralysis
1	10	No movement. Contraction of muscle is palpable or visible.
2	25	Full muscle movement against gravity, with support.
3	50	Normal movement against gravity.
4	75	Normal full movement against gravity and against minimal resistance.
5	100	Normal strength. Normal full movement against gravity and against full resistance.

NORMAL RANGE OF JOINT MOTION

Joint Movement	Normal Range (Degrees)
Shoulders	
Abduction: Moves arm laterally from side position to above head, palm facing outermost	180
Elbow	
Flexion: Brings lower arm forward and upward toward shoulder	150
Wrist	
Flexion: Brings fingers of hand toward inner part of forearm	80–90
Extension: Straightens wrist from flexed position	80–90
Hyperextension: Bends fingers back as far as wrist permits	70–90
Abduction: Bends wrist to thumb side while palm faces upward	0–20
Adduction: Bends wrist toward fifth finger side, palm facing upward	30–50
Hand and finger	
Flexion: Makes a fist	90
Extension: Straightens fingers	90
Hyperextension: Bends fingers and hand back ar far as possible	30
Abduction: Spreads fingers apart	20
Adduction: Brings fingers together from abducted position	20

Neurologic: **Mental status:** Alert, oriented to time, place, person, and situation. Remote and recent memory intact. Coordinated movements, upright posture, steady gait and balance. **Cranial nerves:** Nerves I to XII intact. **Sensory:** Feels and identifies correct location of soft touch bilaterally. Ability to identify tastes accurately.

Anus and Rectum: Ability to contract anal sphincter. Rectal examination negative for masses or lesions.

Genitalia: Penis not tender; no discharge or lesions. Testes not tender; no pitting. Negative for inguinal and femoral hernias. No vaginal discharge.

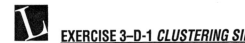

EXERCISE 3–D-1 _CLUSTERING SIMILAR DATA USING A BODY SYSTEMS MODEL_

In the spaces below, cluster the data from the scenario about Mr. Lopez.

Integumentary

Subjective Data _____

_____

Objective Data _____

_____

Respiratory

Subjective Data _____

_____

Objective Data _____

_____

Cardiovascular

Subjective Data _____

_____

Objective Data _____

_____

Neurologic

Subjective Data _____

_____

Objective Data _____

_____

Musculoskeletal

Subjective Data _____

_____

Objective Data _____

_____

Gastrointestinal

Subjective Data _____

_____

Objective Data _____

_____

Genitourinary

Subjective Data _____

_____

Objective Data _____

_____

Reproductive

Subjective Data _____

_____

Objective Data _____

_____

Endocrine

Subjective Data _____

_____

Objective Data _____

_____

Psychiatric/Psychologic

Subjective Data _____

_____

Objective Data _____

_____

Current health promotion practices

Subjective Data _____

_____

Objective Data _____

_____

Home situation and relationship with others

Subjective Data _____

_____

Objective Data _____

_____

Correct responses are on p. 30.

Functional Health Patterns

During assessment, the nurse collects data for each functional health pattern. The following list cites examples of clustered subjective and objective data related to each pattern. The list is not inclusive (see Case Study #1, Chapter 8).

PATTERN #1: HEALTH PERCEPTION AND HEALTH MANAGEMENT

The client's perception and management of health and well-being.

Subjective Data	Objective Data
• Reason for admission (visit)	• Use of illicit drugs
• Prescription and nonprescription medications	• Height and weight

PATTERN #2: NUTRITIONAL AND METABOLIC

Describes dietary intake; fluid and electrolyte balance; condition of skin, hair, and nails.

Subjective Data	Objective Data
• Appetite; caffeine use	• Prescribed diet
• Food preferences	• Percentage of food eaten (inpatient); outpatient diet diary
• Allergies	

PATTERN #3: ELIMINATION

Describes patterns of excretory function of the bowel, bladder, and skin.

Subjective Data	Objective Data
Bladder	
• Frequency, nocturia	• Urine amount, color, odor
• Usual characteristics of urine output	• Specific gravity
Bowel	
• Frequency and usual characteristics of stool	• Stool amount, color, consistency
Skin	
• Excess perspiration	• Diaphoresis

PATTERN #4: ACTIVITY AND EXERCISE

Describes pattern of exercise and activity and respiratory and circulatory function.

Subjective Data	Objective Data
Breathing	
• Shortness of breath (SOB) or pain with exercise	• Respiratory rate, depth, rhythm
Circulation	
• Family history of heart disease	• Apical rate, rhythm
	• Blood pressure
	• Peripheral pulses

Mobility

• Usual exercise pattern	• Range of motion (ROM)
• Leisure activities	• Strength, posture

PATTERN #5: SLEEP AND REST

Describes patterns of sleep and rest and perception of energy level.

Subjective Data	Objective Data
• Usual hours of sleep	• Observe time of sleep and naps
	• Sleep aids; frequent yawning

PATTERN #6: COGNITIVE AMD PERCEPTUAL

Describes patterns of hearing, vision, taste, touch, smell, pain perception, language, memory, and decision making.

Subjective Data	Objective Data
• Sensory and perceptual problems: hearing, vision, touch, smell taste	• Ability see, hear smell, feel
	• Seizure activity

PATTERN #7: SELF-PERCEPTION AND SELF-CONCEPT

Describes attitudes about self and perceived abilities.

Subjective Data	Objective Data
• Attitudes about self	• Body posture
• Impact of illness on self	• Eye contact

PATTERN #8: ROLE AND RELATIONSHIP

Describes effectiveness of roles and relationships with significant others.

Subjective Data	Objective Data
• Employment interaction	• Observed

PATTERN #9: SEXUALITY AND REPRODUCTIVE

Describes actual or perceived satisfaction or problems with sexuality.

Subjective Data	Objective Data
• Impact illness on sexuality	• Breast self examination
• Mammogram	
• Menstrual history; children	• Testicular exam

PATTERN #10: COPING AND STRESS TOLERANCE

Describes ability to manage stress and use of support systems.

Subjective Data	Objective Data
• Stressors in past year	• Interactions with family
• Usual coping methods	
• Support system	

PATTERN #11: VALUE AND BELIEF

Describes religious, spiritualy, value, and belief system.

Subjective Data	Objective Data
• Religion; spirituality	• Requests visit with chaplain
• Expresses concern with meaning of belief and death	• Signed advance directive
	• Questions moral and ethical implications of therapeutic regimen

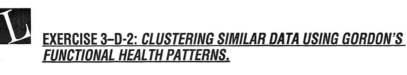

EXERCISE 3–D-2: _CLUSTERING SIMILAR DATA USING GORDON'S FUNCTIONAL HEALTH PATTERNS._

In the spaces below, cluster the data from scenario about Mr. Lopez.

1. Health Perception-Health Management Pattern

Subjective Data _____

_____

Objective Data _____

_____

2. Nutritional-Metabolic Pattern

Subjective Data _____

_____

Objective Data _____

_____

3. Elimination Pattern

Subjective Data _____

_____

Objective Data _____

_____

4. Activity-Exercise Pattern

Subjective Data _____

_____

Objective Data _____

_____

5. **Sleep-Rest Pattern**

Subjective Data _____

_____

Objective Data _____

_____

6. **Cognitive-Perceptual Pattern**

Subjective Data _____

_____

Objective Data _____

_____

7. **Self-Perception and Self-Concept Pattern**

Subjective Data _____

_____

Objective Data _____

_____

8. **Role-Relationships Pattern**

Subjective Data _____

_____

Objective Data _____

_____

9. **Sexuality-Reproductive Pattern**

Subjective Data _____

_____

Objective Data _____

_____

10. **Coping-Stress Tolerance Pattern**

Subjective Data _____

_____

Objective Data _____

_____

11. **Value-Belief Pattern**

Subjective Data _____

_____

Objective Data _____

_____

Correct responses are on p. 31

■ REASSESSMENT OF CLIENTS

When does reassessment occur? Who performs the reassessment? How frequently is reassessment conducted? Reassessment is a review process that is ongoing throughout the client's contact with the organization. The interval between reassessments is defined in the health care organization's policies for inpatient, outpatient, nursing home, home care, and other settings.

Reassessment may occur at a return appointment to an ambulatory care clinic, throughout an inpatient hospital stay, and at a follow-up home visit. An organization's policies indicate time frames and criteria for reassessment. For example, an organization may require reassessments every 8 hours for inpatients and reassessments at each clinic visit.

Clients are reassessed at specified times throughout a client's course of treatment to determine the client's response to treatment when a significant change occurs in the client's condition when a significant change occurs in the client's diagnosis.

■ REPORTING AND RECORDING THE ASSESSMENT AND REASSESSMENT DATA

How are the data reported? Where are the data recorded to ensure the continuum of care? (See Chapter 6, Documentation)

Continuity of care is facilitated by reporting and recording specific information relevant to the client's therapeutic regimen. The interdisciplinary team members are responsible and accountable for documenting the care rendered. The interdisciplinary team members document their interventions and the client's response in the medical record. Team members read each others' notes to gain an understanding of the client's progress in meeting outcomes. The current trend is to document assessment and reassessment data on preprinted or computerized assessment and reassessment medical record forms to ensure uniform collection, recording, and reporting of data by the interdisciplinary team. Documentation forms may be structured in the format of a medical (such as a body system approach) or a nursing model (for example, functional health patterns).

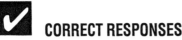 **CORRECT RESPONSES**

EXERCISE 3–A: IDENTIFICATION OF SUBJECTIVE DATA

1. "For the past 2 weeks, I have had to go to the bathroom a lot. I feel a need to hurry to the bathroom. It burns when I pass my water. My lower back hurts."
2. The urine "is dark orange."
3. The urine "smells strong."
4. "I drink three cups of coffee a day and a tall glass of water at night; I only pass a little urine; my skin feels dry."
5. "I get dizzy when I stand up."

EXERCISE 3–B IDENTIFICATION OF OBJECTIVE DATA.

1. Cloudy, thick urine
2. Oral temperature 38.0° C (100.4° F)
3. Urine culture revealed the presence of *Escherichia coli.*
4. Dark amber urine.
5. Foul-smelling urine

6. Daily fluid intake of 780 mL
7. Skin tented and returned to normal shape in 10 seconds
8. Specific gravity >1.030
9. Lying BP 130/80; standing BP 110/70; pulse 90

EXERCISE 3–C DATA VALIDATION

1. Client data

Subjective "For the past 2 weeks, I have had to go to the bathroom a lot; I feel a need to hurry to the bathroom. It burns when I pass my water. My lower back hurts."

Objective Cloudy, thick urine; oral temperature 38.0°C (100.4°F); urine culture revealed the presence of *Escherichia coli.*

Normal value Transparent, clear liquid; urine culture reveals no microorganisms; oral temperature 37.0°C (98.6°F)

2. Client data

Subjective Urine "is dark orange."

Objective Dark amber urine

Normal value Straw-, amber-colored;

3. Client data

Subjective Urine "smells strong."

Objective Foul-smelling urine.

Normal value Faint aromatic odor

4. Client data

Subjective "I drink three cups of coffee a day and a tall glass of water at night; I only pass a little urine."

Objective Daily fluid intake of 780 mL; specific gravity >1.030; pulse 90; skin tented and returned to normal shape in 10 seconds.

Normal value Normal 24-hour fluid intake for an adult is 1500 mL; the normal total fluid intake in 24 hours is 2500 mL, with the additional 1000 mL acquired from foods and oxidation of these foods; when skin turgor is tested, skin returns to normal shape immediately; specific gravity 1.010 to 1.025.

5. Client data

Subjective "I get dizzy when I stand up."

Objective Lying BP 130/80; standing BP 110/70; pulse 90

Normal value BP for adult male 120/80; pulse rate for adult is 80 with a range 60 to 100

EXERCISE 3–D-1: CLUSTERING OF THE DATA USING A BODY SYSTEMS MODEL

1. Integumentary

Subjective Data "I drink three cups of coffee a day and a tall glass of water at night; I only pass a little urine; my skin feels dry."

Objective Data Skin tented and returned to normal shape in 10 seconds; daily fluid intake is 780 mL.

2. Respiratory

Subjective Data None expressed by client

Objective Data In no acute distress

3. Cardiovascular

Subjective Data

"Dizzy when I stand up"

Objective Data

Lying BP 130/80; standing BP 110/70; pulse 90

4. Nervous

Subjective Data None expressed by client

Objective Data No abnormal data observed

5. Musculoskeletal

Subjective Data None expressed by client

Objective Data No abnormal data observed

6. Gastrointestinal

Subjective Data None expressed by client

Objective Data No abnormal data observed

7. Genitourinary

Subjective Data "For the past 2 weeks, I have had to go to the bathroom a lot; I feel a need to hurry to the bathroom; it burns when I pass my water; urine "smells strong"; urine is a "dark orange."

Objective Data Urine foul smelling, dark amber, cloudy, thick; specific gravity >1.030; *Escherichia coli* present in urine culture; oral temperature 38.0°C (100.4°F).

8. Reproductive

Subjective Data None expressed by client

Objective Data No abnormal data observed

9. Endocrine

Subjective Data <u>None expressed by client</u>

Objective Data <u>No abnormal data noted</u>

10. Psychiatric/Psychologic

Subjective Data <u>None expressed by client</u>

Objective Data <u>No abnormal data noted</u>

11. Current health promotion practices

Subjective Data <u>"I drink three cups of coffee a day and a tall glass of water at night . . ."</u>

Objective Data <u>Yearly physical and dental examinations; received yearly immunization for influenza and a pneumococcal vaccine 2 years ago. 24-hour fluid intake <2500 mL</u>

12. Home situation and relationship with others

Subjective Data <u>"We are a very close family, and every Sunday we attend the Catholic church in our neighborhood."</u>

Objective Data <u>Married 42 years; one child lives with parents; other children work in the restaurant; children live in parents' neighborhood.</u>

EXERCISE 3–D-2: CLUSTERING DATA USING GORDON'S 11 FUNCTIONAL HEALTH PATTERNS

1. Health Perception-Health Management Pattern

Subjective Data <u>"For the past 2 weeks, I have had to go to the bathroom a lot."</u>

Objective Data <u>Yearly physical and dental appointments; yearly influenza immunization and pneumococcal vaccine 2 years ago.</u>

2. Nutritional-Metabolic Pattern

Subjective Data <u>"I drink three cups of coffee a day and a tall glass of water at night; I only pass a little urine."</u>

Objective Data <u>Daily fluid intake 780 mL; skin turgor revealed tenting and skin returned to nor-</u>

mal shape in 10 seconds; specific gravity >1.030

3. Elimination Pattern

Subjective Data <u>"For the past 2 weeks, I have had to go to the bathroom a lot; I feel a need to hurry to the bathroom; it burns when I pass my water; the urine "smells strong and is dark orange."</u>

Objective Data <u>Dark-amber urine; foul-smelling, cloudy, and thick urine; oral temperature 38.0°C (100.4°F); urine culture revealed *Escherichia coli.*</u>

4. Activity-Exercise Pattern

Subjective Data <u>"I get dizzy when I stand up."</u>

Objective Data <u>Lying BP 130/80; standing BP 110/70; pulse 90</u>

5. Sleep-Rest Pattern

Subjective Data <u>None expressed by the client.</u>

Objective Data <u>No abnormal data collected or observed.</u>

6. Cognitive-Perceptual Pattern

Subjective Data <u>None verbalized by client.</u>

Objective Data <u>No abnormal data observed.</u>

7. Self-Perception and Self-Concept Pattern

Subjective Data <u>None expressed by client.</u>

Objective Data <u>No abnormal data observed.</u>

8. Role-Relationship Pattern

Subjective Data <u>"My wife . . . is a good woman and raised our five children while I got our restaurant started. We are a very close family . . . ."</u>

Objective Data <u>No abnormal data observed.</u>

9. Sexuality-Reproductive Pattern

Subjective Data <u>None expressed by client.</u>

Objective Data <u>No abnormal data observed.</u>

10. Coping-Stress Tolerance Pattern

Subjective Data <u>None expressed by client.</u>

Objective Data <u>In no acute distress</u>

11. Value-Belief Pattern

Subjective Data <u>" . . . each Sunday we attend the Catholic church in our neighborhood."</u>

Objective Data <u>No requests for spiritual or religious support during clinic visit.</u>

Diagnosis: Identifying a Problem or Deficit

To establish the cause of a client's illness, the interdisciplinary health care team uses scientific methods to evaluate the history of the disease process, the subjective and objective data, laboratory data, and special tests. The value of establishing a diagnosis is to provide a logical basis for treatment and prognosis.

To identify nursing diagnoses, nurses analyze data (look at the separate pieces), and synthesize (put together) similar pieces. A composite picture is developed and nursing diagnoses formulated based on the response of clients to changes in health status and the nurses' ability to help find solutions.

The merged or clustered data are grouped in frameworks such as functional health patterns or body systems. In the clinical setting, medical diagnoses and nursing diagnoses are listed as problems in the client's medical record, nursing care plan, and interdisciplinary plan of care.

After medical and nursing diagnoses are identified, priorities of care are established before the remaining phases of the problem-solving approach are initiated. Nursing diagnoses provide a foundation for establishing outcome criteria for nursing care and determining the interventions required to achieve the outcomes.

■ BACKGROUND AND RATIONALE FOR NURSING DIAGNOSES

In 1973, the North American Nursing Diagnosis Association (NANDA) was founded. At that time, nursing leaders were striving to clarify nurses' role in the de-livery of health care. Nursing diagnosis was accepted as the term that described problems identified in nursing practice that were within the realm of nursing to treat. Labels provide a name for the identified problems of clients. In naming clinical phenomena in the form of nursing diagnoses, nurses share a common language to compare and contrast outcomes achieved by particular nursing actions within different settings and populations. Nursing diagnosis emerged as step two of the nursing process and is phase two of the problem-solving approach.

A need to organize nursing diagnoses into an orderly structure evolved with an increase in the number developed and validated. Thus, NANDA generated a taxonomy to classify nursing diagnoses. Taxonomy provides a vocabulary for classifying phenomena in the nursing discipline.

A taxonomy is an orderly classification system used in science. NANDA defines classification as "a systematic arrangement in groups or categories according to established criteria; an arrangement of phenomena into groups based on their relationships" (NANDA, 1994a, p. 7).

Nine Human Response Patterns (listed below) serve as the framework for classifying nursing diagnostic labels. For example, in the first human response pattern, Choosing, the nursing diagnostic label is Selection of Alternatives. The diagnostic labels and subsequent definitions facilitate consistency, communication, and utilization of the NANDA taxonomy around the world. NANDA's Nursing Diagnosis Taxonomy I (Appendix A) was accepted by the 1986 General Assembly of NANDA.

Definitions of NANDA'S Human Response Patterns (Appendix A lists nursing diagnoses under each pattern)

Choosing: Selection of alternatives
To select between alternatives; the action of selecting or exercising preference in regard to a matter in which one is a free agent; to determine in favor of a course; to decide in accordance with inclinations.

Communicating: Sending messages
To converse; to impart, confer, or transmit thoughts, feelings, or information, internally or externally, verbally or nonverbally.

Exchanging: Mutual giving and receiving
To give, replenish, or lose something while receiving something in return; the substitution of one element for another; the reciprocal act of giving and receiving.

Feeling: Subjective awareness of information
To experience consciousness, sensation, apprehension, or sense; to be consciously or emotionally affected by a fact, event, or state.

Knowing: Meaning associated with information
To recognize or acknowledge a thing of a person; to be familiar with by experience or through information or report; to be cognizant of something through observation, inquiry, or information; to be conversant with a body of facts, prinicples, or methods of action; to understand.

Moving: Activity
To change the place or position of a body or any member of the body; to put and/or keep in motion; to provoke an excretion or discharge; the urge to action or to do something; to take action.

Perceiving: Reception of information
To apprehend with the mind; to become aware of by the senses; to apprehend what is not open or present to observation; to take in fully or adequately.

Relating: Establishing bonds
To connect; to establish a link between; to stand in some association to another thing, person, or place; to be born or thrust in between things.

Valuing: Assigning of relative worth
To be concerned about; to care; the worth or worthiness; the relative status of a thing, or the esteem in which it is held, according to its real or supposed worth, usefulness, or importance; one's opinion of linking for a real person or thing; to equate in importance.

Source: North American Nursing Diagnosis Association. (1991). In R. M. Carroll-Johnson (Ed.). *Classification of nursing diagnoses: proceeding of the ninth conference.* PA: Lippincott, p. 464.

Professional nursing organizations continue to promote and support NANDA's research and development of nursing diagnoses. Every 2 years NANDA reviews and approves nursing diagnoses that have been researched and tested clinically for their inclusion in the NANDA list of approved diagnostic labels. The American Nurses Association (ANA) supports nursing diagnoses. The *ANA Standards of Clinical Nursing Practice* (1991), Standard II states, "The nurse analyzes assessment data in determining diagnoses." The ANA Social Policy (ANA, 1980, p. 9) statement says, "Nursing is the diagnosis and treatment of human responses to actual or potential health problems." The ANA acknowledged NANDA as the association to be used by the ANA practice councils for the development, review, and approval of nursing diagnoses.

At present there is a movement by nurses to gain reimbursement for nursing interventions. The goal is to identify nursing interventions consistently associated with a nursing diagnosis and to seek reimbursement for those nursing interventions. Reimbursement will lead to true autonomy of the nursing profession. For example, many community health nurses receive third-party reimbursement for nursing interventions rendered to the client.

■ DEFINITIONS OF NURSING DIAGNOSES

Nursing Diagnosis: Nursing diagnosis is a clinical judgment about individual, family, or community responses to actual and potential health problems and life processes. Nursing diagnoses provide the basis for selection of nursing interventions to achieve outcomes for which the nurse is accountable (Approved by the membership at the North American Nursing Diagnosis Association, Ninth Conference, March 1990).

Actual Nursing Diagnosis: Describes human responses to health condition or life processes that exist in an individual, family, or community. It is supported by defining characteristics (manifestations, signs, and symptoms) that cluster in patterns of related cues or inferences (NANDA, 1994a, p. 102).

Risk Nursing Diagnosis: Describes human responses to health conditions or life processes that may develop in a vulnerable individual, family, or community. It is supported by risk factors that contribute to increased vulnerability (NANDA, 1994a, p. 102).

Wellness Nursing Diagnosis: Describes human responses to levels of wellness in an individual, family, or community that have a potential for enhancement to a higher state (NANDA, 1994a, p. 102).

■ COMPONENTS OF A NURSING DIAGNOSIS
(NANDA, 1994a, pp. 102–103)

Label: Provides a name for a problem. It is a concise term or phrase that represents a pattern of related cues. It may include qualifiers (acute, altered, chronic, decreased).

Definition: Provides a clear, precise description, delineates its meaning, and helps differentiate it from similar diagnoses. The definition is not written in the medical record.

Related factors: Conditions or circumstances that contribute to the development or maintenance of a nursing diagnosis.

or

Risk factors: Environmental factors and physiologic, psychologic, genetic, or chemical elements that increase the vulnerability of an individual, family, or community to an unhealthful event.

Defining characteristics: Observable cues and inferences that cluster as manifestations of a nursing diagnosis. These are listed for actual and wellness diagnoses. A defining characteristic is described as "critical" if it must be present to make the diagnosis; the characteristic is described as "major" if it is usually present when the diagnosis exists; is described as "minor" if it provides supporting evidence for the diagnosis but may not be present. Critical and major defining characteristics need to be substantiated by research. "Major defining characteristics are present in 80% to 100% of the clients experiencing the diagnosis and minor as present in 50% to 79% of the clients experiencing the diagnosis" (NANDA, 1994a, p. 12).

QUALIFIERS FOR DIAGNOSES (NANDA, 1994a, p. 104)

Acute:	severe but of short duration
Altered:	a change from baseline
Chronic:	lasting a long time, recurring, habitual, constant
Decreased:	lessened, lesser in size, amount, or degree
Deficient:	inadequate in amount, quality, or degree; defective; not sufficient; incomplete
Depleted:	emptied wholly or in part, exhausted of
Disturbed:	agitated, interrupted, interfered with
Dysfunctional:	abnormal, incomplete functioning
Excessive:	characterized by an amount or quantity that is greater than necessary, desirable, or useful
Increase:	greater in size, amount, or degree
Impaired:	made worse, weakened, damaged, reduced, deteriorated
Ineffective:	not producing the desired effect
Intermittent:	stopping or starting again at intervals, periodic, cyclic
Potential for:	(use with wellness diagnoses)
Enhanced:	made greater, to increase in quality or become more desired

Putting it all together, the following explanations clarify the relationship of the parts of a nursing diagnosis.

Label

What changes have occurred in the client's health? **The first component of a nursing diagnosis is the label (problem).** Labels describe alterations in the client's health status, and the problem is expressed in two to three words (for example, Impaired skin integrity). Alterations cause problems and untoward changes in the client's ability to function. Labels accepted for use in practice are listed alphabetically on the NANDA 1994 Approved Nursing Diagnostic Category list (Appendices A and B). The nurse's accuracy in identifying the problem is vital. Expected outcomes are based on the problem, with subsequent evaluation of outcome attainment.

If nurses encounter difficulties identifying a label, information gaps may exist. In that case, the nurse reassesses the client for further data. The label should be compatible with medical diagnoses and problems and deficits identified by other health care disciplines. Nursing diagnoses may be grouped according to a framework, such as Gordon's Functional Health Patterns, body systems, and NANDA's Human Response Patterns.

The following are examples of NANDA labels: *Activity intolerance* and *Ineffective airway clearance;* they will be discussed throughout the remainder of this book.

NANDA labels
Label: *Activity intolerance*
Label: *Ineffective airway clearance*

Definition

Definitions (see Appendix B) delineate the meaning of the NANDA labels and assist the nurse in selecting the appropriate label that clearly identifies the client's problem. The definitions are not written into the nursing diagnosis. The following are examples of definitions for the labels cited above:

Label: *Activity intolerance*
Definition: A state in which an individual has insufficient physiologic or psychologic energy to

endure or complete required or desired daily activities (NANDA, 1994a, p. 61).

Label: *Ineffective airway clearance*

Definition: A state in which an individual is unable to clear secretions or obstructions from the respiratory tract to maintain airway patency (NANDA, 1994a, p. 26).

Related Factors or Risk Factors (Etiology)

What are the causes of the changes in the client's health status? **The second component of a nursing diagnosis is related factors or risk factors reflecting the etiology causes of the changes in the client's health status.** The cause may be attributed to client's behaviors; pathophysiologic, psychosocial, situational changes in life-style; developmental age; cultural and environmental factors. The phrase *related to (R/T)* serves to connect the label (problem) with the causes of the problem. Related factors are conditions or circumstances that influence the nurse in developing or maintaining a nursing diagnosis (NANDA, 1994, p. 103). Risk factors are environmental factors and physiologic, psychologic, genetic, or chemical elements that increase the vulnerability of an individual, family, or community to an unhealthful event (NANDAa, 1994, p. 103). The related factors are the basis for interventions to resolve the problem.

The use of labels is applicable to all areas of nursing such as medical and surgical, maternity, pediatrics, psychiatry, and community health. The causes of a client's problem, however, may differ from one client to another. For example, *Activity intolerance* (problem) related to immobility (cause) may be the diagnostic statement for an adult with a stroke, and *Activity intolerance* (problem) related to imbalance between oxygen supply and demand (cause) may be the diagnostic statement for a child with congenital heart disease. Another example is *Ineffective airway clearance* (problem) related to altered level of consciousness (cause), which may be the diagnostic statement for an adult with a stroke, and *Ineffective airway clearance* (problem) related to decreased energy level (cause) may be the diagnostic statement for a child with congenital heart disease.

There are numerous causes of clients' problems. Nurses select specific causes that are the basis for the clients' problem. The causes can be influenced by nursing interventions. In Appendix B, related factors and risk factors are grouped for each label.

The following are examples of causes that may be related to clients who demonstrate *Activity intolerance* or *Ineffective airway clearance*. A complete list of related factors are located in Appendix B.

LABEL (PROBLEM): *ACTIVITY INTOLERANCE*
Possible related factors:

1. Immobility
2. Generalized weakness
3. Imbalance between oxygen supply and demand
4. Sedentary life style
5. Bedrest

■ **Stroke Client**

The nurse selected *immobility* as the cause of the client's problem.

Activity intolerance (problem) related to *immobility* (cause).

■ **Client with Congenital Heart Dysfunction**

The nurse selected imbalance between oxygen supply and demand as the cause of the client's problem.

Activity intolerance (problem) related to imbalance between oxygen supply and demand (cause).

LABEL: *INEFFECTIVE AIRWAY CLEARANCE*
Possible causes related to the problem:

1. Decreased energy and fatigue level
2. Obstruction
3. Tracheobronchial infection
4. Trauma
5. Secretions
6. Perceptual or cognitive impairment

■ **Stroke Client**

The nurse selected *altered level of consciousness* as the cause of the client's problem.

Ineffective airway clearance (problem) related to *altered level of consciousness* (cause).

■ **Client with Congenital Heart Dysfunction**

The nurse selected *decreased energy level* as the cause of the client's problem.

Ineffective airway clearance (problem) related to *decreased energy level* (cause).

Defining Characteristics

What observable cues (signs and symptoms) provide evidence to support the selection of a label? **Defining characteristics (signs and symptoms) are observable cues or inferences that, when clustered, provide evidence that a problem exists.** They are included in actual and wellness diagnoses. A defining characteristic is described as critical if it *must* be present to make the diagnosis and is described as major if it is *usually* present when the diagnosis exists. It is described as minor if it provides supporting evidence for the diagnosis but may not be present. Critical and major defining characteristics are substantiated by research (NANDA, 1994a, p. 103).

The defining characteristics are a cluster of clinical cues that describe the behaviors, signs, and symptoms that represent a nursing diagnosis. The defining characteristics provide evidence that a health problem exists. The symptoms (subjective data) are changes that the client feels and expresses verbally to the nurse. The signs (objective data) are observable changes in the client's health status.

Use the phrase *as evidenced by (AEB)* to connect the related factors to the defining characteristics. The defining characteristics provide sufficient evidence to support the nursing diagnosis.

Avoid basing a nursing diagnosis on one item of data. Identify a minimum of three signs and three symptoms to provide sufficient evidence to support the selection of a nursing diagnosis.

Defining characteristics based on the labels, *Activity intolerance* and *Ineffective airway clearance.*

■ **Stroke Client**

Label: *Activity intolerance*

Related to: immobility

Defining Characteristics: as evidenced by verbal report of fatigue or weakness; abnormal heart rate or blood pressure in response to activity; exertional discomfort or dyspnea; electrocardiographic changes reflecting arrhythmias or ischemia.

Example of defining characteristics for the label, *Activity intolerance:*

SUBJECTIVE	OBJECTIVE
"I am too weak to walk."	Unable to walk 5 feet
"I feel fatigued."	Pulse 100 on exertion
"I feel short of breath."	Respiration 28, labored

■ **Client with Congenital Heart Dysfunction**

Label: *Ineffective airway clearance*

Related to: imbalance between oxygen supply and demand

Defining characteristics: as evidenced by

SUBJECTIVE DATA	OBJECTIVE DATA
"I cannot breathe."	Respirations 30, shallow
"I feel plugged up."	Crackling sounds right lower lobe (RLL)
"I cannot cough."	Inability cough up sputum

■ WRITING A NURSING DIAGNOSIS IN THE MEDICAL RECORD

A nursing diagnosis describes the health status of the client and factors contributing to that status. A nursing diagnosis is written by a nurse for problems identified and reflects actual or high-risk problems that require resolution.

An **actual** nursing diagnosis denotes a deviation (Activity intolerance) from normal health status. In writing a nursing diagnosis in the clinical setting, it is easy to remember the PRS components of an actual nursing diagnosis: P = problem; R = related to; S = signs and symptoms.

Usually the entire three-part nursing diagnosis is written out initially in the medical record (plan of care), and subsequent documentation may reflect use of the label only (activity intolerance), a descriptive note of the interventions implemented, and the client's response to the plan of care (inability to walk 5 feet).

■ **Stroke Client: Three-Part Nursing Diagnosis**

Activity intolerance (label) related to immobility (cause) as evidenced by verbal expressions of fatigue, inability to walk 5 feet, pulse 100 on exertion (defining characteristics).

■ **Client with Congenital Heart Dysfunction: Three-Part Nursing Diagnosis**

Ineffective airway clearance (label) related to imbalance between oxygen supply and demand (cause) as evidenced by verbal expressions of shortness of breath, crackling sounds in the right lower lobe, respirations 30 and shallow (defining characteristics).

A **high-risk** nursing diagnosis denotes the presence of risk factors that may cause an actual health problem in the future. At the time of the nurse's initial assessment, the client has not demonstrated defining characteristics to support the formulation of an actual nursing diagnosis; therefore a high-risk nursing diagnosis is formulated. The nursing and interdisciplinary team's interventions are directed at reducing risk factors. A high-risk nursing diagnosis is a two-part statement:

1. high risk label (potential problem)
2. related to (potential cause).

EXAMPLE OF A TWO-PART HIGH-RISK NURSING DIAGNOSIS:

■ **Stroke Client: Two-Part High Risk Nursing Diagnosis**
High risk for injury (potential problem) related to muscle weakness (potential cause).

■ **Client with Congenital Heart Dysfunction: Two-Part High Risk Nursing Diagnosis**
High risk for infection (potential problem) related to reduced body defenses (potential cause)

For a wellness diagnosis, write a one-part statement. The label, "Potential for enhanced" is placed before the words that describe the area that is to be improved, for example, potential for enhanced breastfeeding. When healthy clients indicate a desire to achieve a higher level of functioning, wellness diagnoses are formulated. Nurses in community health settings find the wellness diagnoses useful to meet the needs of the client population served. In acute care settings, the plan of care usually addresses actual and high-risk diagnoses, which are considered of primary importance at that time rather than wellness diagnoses. However, with the increased focus on primary care, nurse-managed health promotion clinics present an opportunity for nursing to promote wellness diagnoses such as *Health-seeking behaviors.*

■ MEDICAL DIAGNOSES

In collaborative practice, it is important for nurses to know the perspective of other professions, just as they need to understand the nursing perspective. Plans of care should reflect nursing and medical diagnoses. Traditionally, medical diagnoses (such as diabetes mellitus) have been derived by physicians after taking the initial history and conducting the physical examination. A medical diagnosis identifies a disease process or pathologic condition, and the diagnosis guides the therapeutic regimen. Through the years, other health care team members (nurse practitioners; psychologists) have used medical diagnoses in identifying a client's problem.

A medical diagnosis does not necessarily consider the human responses to the pathologic condition (for example, denial of diabetes mellitus). As long as the disease process is present, the medical diagnosis does not change. However, the nursing diagnosis changes as the client's response changes. For a newly diagnosed noncompliant diabetic client, a nurse may initially formulate the nursing diagnosis, *Noncompliance with diabetic regimen related to knowledge deficit as evidenced by incorrect administration of insulin, failure to follow prescribed diet, and failure to perform proper foot care.* Subsequent to a nurse's reinforcment of the initial teaching, the medical diagnosis remains the same; however, the nursing diagnosis changes to reflect that as the client gains knowledge of the diabetic regimen, the client's compliance increases and the problem decreases.

EXERCISE 4–A:

Formulation of a Nursing Diagnostic Statement. Formulate and write nursing diagnoses for Mr. Lopez in the scenario in Chapter 3.

1. Label: _____

   Related to: _____

   Defining characteristics (as evidenced by): _____
   _____
   _____
   _____

2. Label: _____

   Related to: _____

   Defining characteristics (as evidenced by): _____
   _____
   _____
   _____

3. Label: _____

   Related to: _____

   Defining characteristics (as evidenced by): _____
   _____
   _____
   _____
   _____

4. Label: _____

   Related to: _____

   Defining characteristics (as evidenced by):
   _____
   _____
   _____

Correct responses are on the following page.

✔ **CORRECT RESPONSES**

EXERCISE 4–A. FORMULATION OF A NURSING DIAGNOSTIC STATEMENT

1. Label: <u>Altered urinary elimination</u>

Related to: <u>urinary tract infection</u>

Defining characteristics (as evidenced by): <u>verbal expressions of urgency, burning sensation, passing minimal urine; urine specimen foul-smelling, dark-orange color, cloudy and thick; fluid intake of 780 mL/24 hours, skin remained tented, sp gr ≥1.030.</u>

2. Label: <u>Knowledge deficit</u>

Related to: <u>unfamiliarity with information resources</u>

Defining characteristics (as evidenced by): <u>presence of urinary tract infection for a 2-week period with no evidence of seeking help from health care professionals.</u>

3. Label: <u>Acute pain</u>

Related to: <u>irritation of bladder and urethral mucosa resulting from unresolved urinary tract infection</u>

Defining characteristics (as evidenced by): <u>verbal description of burning sensation upon urination, and low back pain</u>

4. Label: <u>Urge incontinence</u>

Related to: <u>unresolved urinary tract infection</u>

Defining characteristics (as evidenced by): <u>Verbal expression of urgent need to urinate.</u>

Plan of Care and Outcome Identification

The plan of care and identification of outcomes afford nurses, other interdisciplinary team members, clients, family members, significant others, and the community an opportunity to formulate a mutually agreed-upon plan of action aimed at resolving the client's problems. Nursing care plans, interdisciplinary plans of care, and clinical pathways are directed at returning the client to an optimal state of wellness. Nurses and interdisciplinary team members tailor the plans and clinical pathways toward the age-specific (infants and children, young adults, adults, geriatric) and developmental needs of clients.

Plans and pathways include the priority problems of the client, outcomes the client is expected to achieve, and interventions that nurses and the interdisciplinary team will implement to aid the client in attaining the outcomes. Plans and clinical pathways provide evidence that nurses meet ANA Standards III and IV of *Clinical Nursing Practice* (ANA, 1991):

> **Standard III:** Outcome identification. The nurse identifies outcomes individualized to the client.
>
> **Standard IV:** Planning. The nurse develops a plan of care that prescribes interventions to attain expected outcomes.

To facilitate the continuum of care, the nursing staff and interdisciplinary team members address discharge planning needs noted on nursing care plans, interdisciplinary plans of care, and clinical pathways. Discharge planning begins on admission into a health care system and is based on the initial assessment and reassessment of clients. The plans and pathways prepare clients to move from one level of care (for example, inpatient stay) to another level of care (outpatient). For example, outside the hospital, the clients' care may be delivered in their homes, in community nursing homes, or in board-and-care settings.

■ COMPONENTS OF PLAN AND OUTCOME IDENTIFICATION

- Priority ranking of problems
- Establishing measurable outcomes
- Specifying interventions
- Writing care plan or clinical pathway

• Priority Ranking of Problems

What is the urgency of treating each problem? Which problems should be resolved first? When are problems referred to other members of the health care team? During assessment, the nurse encounters a number of client problems. Nurses, the interdisciplinary team, clients, families, and significant others arrange the client's problems in order of their importance and urgency. After the database has been collected and analyzed, the problems are organized in a problem list, with subsequent development of nursing care plans, interdisciplinary plans of care, or clinical pathways.

Problems are needs that clients are unable to meet without assistance from the health care team. Each problem is labeled and numbered for easier identification throughout the medical record and categorized as active or inactive on the problem list. Nursing diagnoses and medical diagnoses are recorded on the problem list located at the beginning of the medical records. A list may contain two or more top-priority problems.

A Problem List

Priority	Date Entered	Date Inactive	Client Problems
1	09/30/97		Ineffective airway clearance
2	09/30/97		Pneumonia
3	09/30/97		Activity intolerance

On the other hand, in nursing care plans, the nursing diagnoses are ranked **high, medium,** or **low** priority. Nurses, clients, and families focus their efforts on resolving the client's high-priority problems first. High-priority problems reflect a life-threatening situation, for example, ineffective airway clearance. Medium-priority problems deal with client needs that are not emergencies and not life-threatening; for example, "requires assistance with a bath." Low-priority problems may not be directly related to the specific illness or prognosis; for example, "needs help with financial problems." A high-priority problem (establishing a clear airway) requires prompt attention, before any is given a low-priority problem (meeting the client's social needs). If a problem is not within the scope of nursing to treat, it is referred to an appropriate health care team member. Clients' medium-to-low priority problems may not be addressed during their hospitalization due to the shorter inpatient stays. In such cases, continuing care may be provided during return visits to outpatient clinics, during nursing home care stay, or by public health agencies, hospice centers, or other health care agencies and settings.

Priorities may change after the initial assessment. For example, a client's initial high-priority nursing diagnosis was *Activity intolerance.* When reassessing the client, the nurse noted that the client complained of shortness of breath; that the client's respirations were 30 and shallow, and there were crackling sounds right lower lobe. The problem of maintaining a clear airway constituted a higher priority than *Activity intolerance;* therefore, with the shift in problems, *Ineffective airway clearance* became the high-priority problem and *Activity intolerance* a medium priority.

Establishing the priority ranking of diagnoses is simplified through the use of Maslow's (1968) Hierarchy of Needs. The hierarchic framework includes physiologic, psychologic, and social needs. The five levels of the hierarchy (Fig. 5–1) are:

- physiologic
- safety and security
- love and belonging
- self-esteem
- self-actualization

Physiologic needs are satisfied before higher-level needs such as self-actualization. For example, a person who lacks food will search for food before seeking fulfillment of career goals.

The following examples describe human needs identified at each level on Maslow's hierarchy of needs model.

■ Physiologic Needs	
Air	Circulation
Water	Rest and mobility
Food	Skin care
Pain avoidance	Rest and mobility
Temperature maintenance	Shelter
Elimination	Sleep

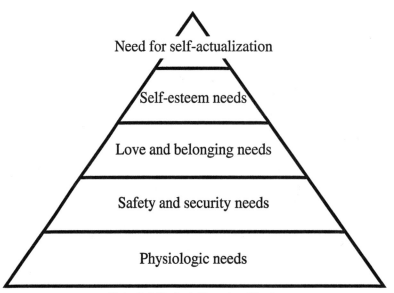

Figure 5–1 Maslow's Hierarchy of Needs

■ **Safety and Security Needs**

No environmental hazards   Clothing
Stable living condition   Protection
Societal rules and laws   Freedom from
No threats real or   infection
   imagined   Freedom from fear

■ **Love and Belonging Needs**

Giving and receiving of   Relationship to
   affection   friends, family,
Affiliation with a group   peers and the
Sexuality   community

■ **Self-esteem Needs**

Feelings of indepen-   Feelings of competence
   dence   Feelings of self-worth
Respect of colleagues   and self-approval

■ **Self-actualization Needs**

All the lower level needs have been met
Fulfillment of life's goals
Content with self and the environment

Stroke Client: Priority Ranking of Nursing Diagnoses

Nursing Diagnosis	Maslow's needs	Ranking
Ineffective airway clearance	Physiologic	High
Activity intolerance	Physiologic	Medium
Potential for injury	Safety/security	Medium

Client with Congenital Heart Dysfunction: Priority Ranking of Nursing Diagnoses

Nursing Diagnosis	Maslow's needs	Ranking
Ineffective airway clearance	Physiologic	High
Activity intolerance	Physiologic	Medium
Potential for injury	Safety	Medium

EXERCISE 5–A: *PRIORITY RANKING OF NURSING DIAGNOSES*

Rank the nursing diagnoses identified for Mr. Lopez in the scenario (Chapter 3) in order of importance, starting with the highest priority (#1) to the lowest priority (#4).

NURSING DIAGNOSIS	MASLOW'S NEEDS	RANKING
1. _____	1. _____	1. _____
2. _____	2. _____	2. _____
3. _____	3. _____	3. _____
4. _____	4. _____	4. _____

Correct responses are on p. 56.

Application of critical thinking in establishing the priority ranking of the diagnoses for Mr. Lopez: Treating the urinary tract infection with antibiotics and increasing the fluid intake will lead to the resolution of the pain and urgency to void. While treating the infection, nurses and other health care team members collaborate to teach clients preventive measures to avoid a recurrence of the infection.

● **Establishing Measurable Outcomes**

What end results measure the resolution of the clients' problems? **Outcomes** are the realistic, measurable goals or objectives the client is expected to achieve. *Goals, objectives, expected outcomes* and *desired client outcomes* are synonyms, meaning the same as *outcomes*. Outcomes represent the yardsticks for measuring the end results of care. That is, doing the right things right leads to successful measurable outcomes. Health care is directed toward achieving outcomes. They are the basis for the nursing care plan, interdisciplinary plan of care, and clinical pathways.

With the trend toward shorter inpatient stays, the interdisciplinary health care team strives to appraise realistically outcomes that can be accomplished in a specified period of time. Outcomes identified by nurses must mesh with the outcomes set by dietitians, physical and occupational therapists, physicians, social workers, and other members of the interdisciplinary team. Outcomes are established with clients, families, and significant others. Nurses and the interdisciplinary team document that the plan and outcomes were discussed with the client, family, and significant others. Individuals' failure to agree with the identified outcomes leads to the identification of unrealistic outcomes, impeding resolution of the problem.

Outcomes are based on the medical and nursing diagnoses. To formulate outcomes, the medical diagnoses and nursing diagnoses are reviewed, and a positive statement is written to resolve the problem identified. One or more outcomes may be written for a medical diagnosis and a nursing diagnosis.

Outcomes identify the steps the client will accomplish in order to achieve the outcomes. Outcomes give direction to nursing and interdisciplinary interventions and provide the foundation for evaluating care. Recognizing the focus on cost-containment measures, the nursing profession can assume the role of an advocate in ensuring the rights of clients to quality care through clearly defined outcomes.

Each outcome includes a **measurable verb** to facilitate the evaluation process. Measurable verbs denote actions that can be seen, heard, or palpated by the nurses and the interdisciplinary team. Outcomes are written on the nursing care plan, interdisciplinary plan of care, or clinical pathway. In the evaluation step of the problem-solving process, the nurse and the interdisciplinary team review the written outcomes to evaluate whether the client has successfully met the outcomes.

Outcome Statement
- Date written
- Subject
- Measurable verbs
- Outcome
- Criteria
- Target time

Subject. **Subject** signals *who* is to achieve the outcome. For example, the client, family, significant others, or community.

■ **Stroke Client: Subject**
Nursing diagnosis: *Activity intolerance*
Date: 9/15/97

1. **Daughter** will describe plan for client's care at home realistically by 9/30/97.
2. **Family friend** will walk client 50 feet every evening by 9/30/97.

■ **Client with Congenital Heart Dysfunction: Subject**
Nursing diagnosis: *Ineffective airway clearance*
Date: 9/15/97

1. **Client** will expectorate lung secretions unassisted by 9/20/97.
2. **Mother** will demonstrate use of oxygen equipment accurately by 9/30/97.

Measurable Verbs. **Measurable verbs** indicate the actions, behaviors, and responses of the client that can be seen, heard, smelled, or felt and, therefore, are measurable. Write measurable verbs in the future tense by prefacing the measurable verb with the transitive verb *will.* For a list of verbs, refer to Appendix E.

■ **Stroke Client: Measurable Verbs**
Nursing diagnosis: *Activity intolerance*
Date: 9/15/97

1. Daughter **will describe** plan for client's care at home realistically by 9/30/97.
2. Family friend **will walk** client 50 feet every evening by 9/30/97.

■ **Client with Congenital Heart Dysfunction: Measurable Verbs**
Nursing diagnosis: *Ineffective airway clearance*
Date: 9/15/97

1. Client **will expectorate** lung secretions un-assisted by 9/20/97.
2. Mother **will demonstrate** use of oxygen equipment accurately by 9/30/97.

Outcome. **Outcomes** indicate the expected physiologic, psychologic, social, and life style responses of clients to interventions.

■ **Stroke Client: Outcomes**
Nursing diagnosis: *Activity intolerance*
Date: 9/15/97

1. Daughter will describe **plan for client care at home** realistically by 9/30/97.
2. Family friend will walk **client 50 feet** every evening by 9/30/97.

■ **Client with Congenital Heart Dysfunction: Outcomes**
Nursing diagnosis: *Ineffective airway clearance*
Date: 9/15/97

1. Client will expectorate **lung secretions** unassisted by 9/20/97.
2. Mother will demonstrate **use of oxygen equipment** accurately by 9/30/97.

Criteria. **Criteria** gauge the client's progress in achieving the outcomes. The criteria indicate the degree of proficiency required to accomplish the end results.

■ **Stroke Client: Criteria**
Nursing diagnosis: *Activity intolerance*
Date: 9/15/97

1. Daughter will describe plan for client care at home **realistically** by 9/30/97.
2. Family friend will walk client 50 feet **every evening** by 9/30/97.

■ **Client with Congenital Heart Dysfunction: Criteria**
Nursing diagnosis: *Ineffective airway clearance*
Date: 9/15/97

1. Client will expectorate lung secretions **unassisted** by 9/20/97.
2. Mother will demonstrate use of oxygen equipment **accurately** by 9/30/97.

Target Time. **Target time** indicates the specific time period desired to achieve the outcome. A time limit assists nurses and the interdisciplinary team in the evaluation step to determine if the outcomes were achieved within the specified time period. If not, a plan to reassess the client and the reestablishment of time frames is undertaken by nurses and the interdisciplinary team.

■ **Stroke Client: Target Times**
Nursing diagnosis: *Activity intolerance*
Date: 9/15/97

1. Daughter will describe plan for client care at home realistically **by 9/30/97.**
2. Family friend will walk client 50 feet every evening **by 9/30/97.**

■ **Client with Congenital Heart Dysfunction: Target Times**
Nursing diagnosis: *Ineffective airway clearance*
Date: 9/15/97

1. Client will expectorate lung secretions unassisted **by 9/20/97.**
2. Mother will demonstrate use of oxygen equipment accurately **by 9/30/97.**

■ **Stroke Client: Outcome Statement**
Client (subject) will employ (measurable verb) safety measures (outcome) willingly (criteria) within 2 days (target time).

■ **Client with Congenital Heart Dysfunction: Outcome Statement**
Mother (subject) will monitor (measurable verb) client's activity level (outcome) daily (criteria) by 9/25/97 (target time).

EXERCISE 5–B: *IDENTIFICATION OF OUTCOMES*

The purpose of Exercise 5–B is to help the student in formulating outcomes. In the spaces below, write outcome for Mr. Lopez in the scenario in Chapter 3.

1. Nursing diagnosis: _____
   Outcome
   Date: _____
   Subject: _____
   Measurable verb: _____
   Outcome: _____
   Criteria: _____
   Target time: _____

2. Nursing diagnosis: _____
   Outcome
   Date: _____
   Subject: _____
   Measurable verb: _____
   Outcome: _____
   Criteria: _____
   Target time: _____

3. Nursing diagnosis: _____
   Outcome
   Date: _____
   Subject: _____
   Measurable verb: _____
   Outcome: _____
   Criteria: _____
   Target time: _____

4. Nursing diagnosis: _____
   Outcome
   Date: _____
   Subject: _____
   Measurable verb: _____
   Outcome: _____
   Criteria: _____
   Target time: _____

Correct responses are on p. 56.

• Specifying Interventions

What actions are implemented by nurses and the interdisciplinary team to assist the client in achieving the outcomes? **Interventions** are specific actions that nurses and the interdisciplinary team implement to assist clients in achieving outcomes. *Nursing interventions, nursing actions,* and *nursing orders* are used interchangeably. They denote specific, measurable, observable, and realistic actions performed by nurses and the interdisciplinary team.

Nursing interventions reduce or resolve the cause of the problem described in the nursing diagnosis. One or more interventions may be written to address a nursing diagnosis. To facilitate continuity of care, nurses discuss applicable interventions with the interdisciplinary team. Subsequently the interventions are written on nursing care plans, interdisciplinary plans of care, and clinical pathways. Nurses and the team record the client's response to the interventions in the progress notes.

A need to identify and generate a list of nursing

interventions evolved with the increased cost of health care, the restructuring of the delivery of care, and the reduction in the work force. Nursing interventions classification (NIC) (McCloskey & Bulechek, 1992) was created to assist practitioners in documenting their care and to facilitate the development of nursing knowledge through the evaluation of client outcomes. Research was conducted to standardize the language used to describe the interventions and devise a system to organize the interventions.

Classifying nursing interventions is "the ordering or arranging of nursing activities into groups or sets on the basis of their relationships and the assigning of intervention labels to these groups" (McCloskey & Bulechek, 1992 p. xvii). Nursing interventions are organized into a taxonomy similar to that used to arrange nursing diagnoses. The classification facilitates clinical testing of nursing interventions, thereby helping to advance nursing knowledge. When using standardized language to document practice, nurses compare and evaluate the effectiveness of care delivered in multiple settings (inpatient units, outpatient units, nursing homes, home care) by different providers (nurse practitioners, critical care nurses, psychiatric nurses). The use of standardized language communicates the essence of nursing care to others as well.

The NIC can be used to determine the cost of services provided by nurses, and it helps to identify interventions proven effective in managing the care of clients with specific diagnoses. Computer programs facilitate the selection of nursing diagnoses and medical diagnoses, outcomes, and interventions as they relate to specific diagnoses.

McCloskey and Bulechek describe nurse-initiated treatments as "interventions initiated by the nurse in response to a nursing diagnosis," and physician-initiated treatments as "interventions initiated by a physician in response to a medical diagnosis but carried out by a nurse in response to a doctor's order" (McClosky & Bulechek, 1992, p. xvii).

The following are examples of NIC intervention labels and definitions (McCloskey & Bulechek, 1992):

Nursing intervention: *Positioning*

Definition: Moving the client or a body part to provide comfort, reduce the risk of skin breakdown, promote skin integrity, and promote healing

Activities (partial list): Provide a firm mattress Position in proper body alignment Provide appropriate back support

Nursing intervention: *Vital signs monitoring*

Definition: Collection and analysis of cardiovascular, respiratory, and body temperature data to determine and prevent complications

Activities (partial list): Monitor blood pressure, pulse, temperature, and respiratory status as appropriate Note trends and wide fluctuations in blood pressure

Auscultate blood pressures in both arms and compare as appropriate

(For a complete listing of nursing interventions, refer to McCloskey & Bulechek, 1992.)

Components of Interventions Written on Care Plans and Pathways

The following are components of interventions the nurses and the interdisciplinary team records on nursing care plans, interdisciplinary plans of care, and clinical pathways:

- Date written
- Measurable verb
- Subject
- Outcome
- Target time
- Signature of interdisciplinary team member(s)

1. The **date** indicating the day, month, and year is written on the nursing care plan, the interdisciplinary plan of care, and clinical pathway by the nurse or interdisciplinary team members.
2. **Measurable verbs** define specific actions by the nurses and interdisciplinary team members (See List of Verbs in Appendix E).
3. **Subject** reflects who will receive the nurses' and interdisciplinary team members' actions, for example, the client, the family, or the community.
4. **Outcome** indicates the intended end result of the nurses' and interdisciplinary team members' actions.
5. **Target time** indicates the period when the nurse and interdisciplinary team are to implement the interventions.
6. **Signatures** of the nurse and interdisciplinary team members verify who wrote the interventions.

Types of Interventions. Interventions can be classified into four major categories: diagnostic, therapeutic, teaching and referral.

Diagnostic interventions assess the progress of the client toward achieving the stated outcomes by direct monitoring of the client's activities. Diagnostic interventions may be used to gather additional information in order to fill information gaps.

> ■ **Stroke Client: Diagnostic Intervention**
> 9/3/97 (date) Assess (measurable verb) client's (subject) range of motion in the upper extremities (outcome) by 9/4/97 (target time). Jolene Vezzetti, RN (signature).

> ■ **Client with Congenital Heart Dysfunction: Diagnostic Intervention**
> 9/3/97 (date) Talk (measurable verb) with wife (subject) to identify fears regarding client's use of oxygen at home (outcome), by 1700 hours today (target time). Jolene Vezzetti, RN (signature).

Therapeutic interventions prescribe actions that directly alleviate, correct, or prevent an exacerbation of the problem.

> ■ **Stroke Client: Therapeutic Intervention**
> 9/3/97 (date) Perform (measurable verb) for client passive range of motion (ROM) to left leg (outcome) four times day (target date). Jolene Vezzetti, RN (signature).

> ■ **Client with Congenital Heart Dysfunction: Therapeutic Intervention**
> 9/3/97 (date) Suction (measurable verb) client's (subject) lung secretions until clear (outcome) as needed (target time). Jolene Vezzetti, RN (signature).

Teaching interventions promote self-care of the client by assisting the individual to acquire new behaviors that facilitate resolution of the problem. Teaching interventions emphasize the active participation of the client in the responsibility for self-care. Teaching inter-

ventions help prepare the client and family for discharge from the health care system and continued care in the home or other settings.

> ■ **Stroke Client: Teaching Intervention**
> 9/3/97 (date) Teach (measurable verb) client (subject) use of walker (outcome) by 9/4/97 (target time). Jolene Vezzetti, RN (signature)

> ■ **Client with Congenital Heart Dysfunction: Teaching Intervention**
> 9/3/97 (date) Demonstrate (measurable verb) to family (subject) tracheal suctioning (outcome) at family, next hospital visit, 9/4/97. Jolene Vezzetti, RN (signature).

Referral interventions emphasize the role of nurses as the coordinators and managers of client care within the health care team. Referrals specify additional consultations needed within or outside the discipline of nursing.

> ■ **Stroke Client: Referral Intervention**
> 9/6/97 Consult (measurable verb) with James Jason, physical therapist (subject), regarding client's progress in using the walker correctly (outcome) by 9/8/97. Jolene Vezzetti, RN (signature)

> ■ **Client with Congenital Heart Dysfunction: Referral Intervention**
> 9/6/97 (date) Refer (measurable verb) mother (subject) to city health department special services for children (outcome) by 9/10/97. Jolene Vezzetti, RN (signature)

ℓ   EXERCISE 5–C: *WRITING NURSING INTERVENTIONS*

In the spaces below, write nursing interventions for the outcomes identified for Mr. Lopez in the scenario (Chapter 3). One or more nursing interventions may be identified for each nursing diagnosis and outcome.

1. Nursing diagnosis: <u>Altered urinary elimination</u>
   Outcome Criterion: <u>Client will demonstrate absence of signs and symptoms of a urinary tract infection as evidenced by negative urine cultures; no complaints of pain, burning, urgency, frequency; straw-colored clear urine within 3 days of initiating antibiotic therapy; and increasing fluid intake to 1500 mL/24 hours.</u>
   a. Nursing intervention
      Date written: _____
      Measurable verb: _____
      Subject: _____
      Outcome: _____
      Target time: _____
      Signature: _____
   b. Nursing intervention
      Date written: _____
      Measurable verb: _____
      Subject: _____
      Outcome: _____
      Target time: _____
      Signature: _____

2. Nursing diagnosis: <u>Pain</u>
   Outcome criterion: <u>Client will urinate without discomfort as evidenced by verbalization of no pain or burning on urination within 24 hours of treatment</u>
   a. Nursing intervention
      Date written: _____
      Measurable verb: _____
      Outcome: _____
      Criterion: _____
      Target time: _____
      Signature: _____
   b. Nursing intervention
      Date written: _____
      Measurable verb: _____
      Outcome: _____
      Criterion: _____
      Target time: _____
      Signature: _____
   c. Nursing intervention
      Date written: _____
      Measurable verb: _____
      Outcome: _____
      Criterion: _____
      Target time: _____
      Signature: _____

3. Nursing diagnosis: <u>Urge incontinence</u>
   Outcome criterion: <u>Client will verbalize no urgency to void as evidenced by no frequent voiding in amounts normal for the client within 3 days of initiating treatment</u>
   Nursing intervention
   Date written: _____
   Measurable verb: _____

Subject: _____

Outcome: _____

Target time: _____

Signature: _____

4. Nursing diagnosis: <u>Knowledge deficit (prevention of urinary infection)</u>

Outcome criterion: <u>Client will verbalize precautionary measures to prevent or reduce the risk of another urinary tract infection accurately at the completion of the present clinic visit and on the follow-up telephone call from the clinic nurse</u>

   a. Nursing intervention

      Date written: _____

      Measurable verb: _____

      Subject: _____

      Outcome: _____

      Target time: _____

      Signature: _____

   b. Nursing intervention

      Date written: _____

      Measurable verb: _____

      Subject: _____

      Outcome: _____

      Target time: _____

      Signature: _____

   c. Nursing intervention

      Date written: _____

      Measurable verb: _____

      Subject: _____

      Outcome: _____

      Target time: _____

      Signature: _____

Correct responses are on p. 56.

• Writing the Nursing Care Plan, Interdisciplinary Plan of Care, or Clinical Pathway

After completing the assessment, diagnosis, plan and outcomes identification nurses and the interdisciplinary team write a nursing care plan, interdisciplinary plan of care (see Appendix L), or clinical pathway to organize the client's care. Care plans and clinical pathways resemble blueprints, that is, carefully designed drawings. They organize information about the health status of clients. A plan is individualized, that is, customized to resolve the client's problems. Upon the client's entering a health care system, a plan may be written on a preprinted, designated health care form or on a computer program.

The current trend in health care practice is to write nursing care plans in collaboration with an interdisciplinary team. The nursing care plan may be a separate document or may be incorporated into an interdisciplinary plan of care or clinical pathway, with identification responsibilities specific to nursing.

When developing a written plan or pathway, the nurse and other health care team members use accepted abbreviations and key phrases rather than complete sentences. The plan, written in black ink, is a permanent part of the client's medical record. A computerized plan of care or clinical pathway, which facilitates rapid access to information relevant to clients, may be used by the nursing service and the interdisciplinary team, and is a permanent part of the client's medical record.

The plans or clinical pathways are reviewed by nurses, the interdisciplinary team, clients, and family when appropriate before care is initiated. At some facilities, registered nurses, in the role of case managers, use the plan to discuss assignments with interdisciplinary team members.

Nurses and the interdisciplinary team evaluate the client's progress toward resolution of problems and achievement of mutually agreed upon outcomes. Nurses and the interdisciplinary team review and revise plans and clinical pathways at timely intervals. For example, nurses review care plans and clinical pathways at each shift in the hospital, and before outpatient clinic visits and home visits. After evaluating the client's progress toward meeting the identified outcomes, nurses and the interdisciplinary team note the date of the revision or review on the plan or clinical pathway.

Well-designed nursing care plans, interdisciplinary plans of care, and clinical pathways serve to:

- facilitate the continuum of care, that is, the progression of clients through the health care system from initial admission to discharge
- organize and coordinate the delivery of care
- increase team communication, organization, and evaluation of care
- serve as a database for:
- making out clinical assignments and allocating time and resources
- distributing resources in a health care center
- performing improvement activities

- identifying nursing's unique contribution to client care

On the other hand, ineffectively designed nursing care plans, interdisciplinary plans of care, or clinical pathways lead to failure to:

- fill information gaps
- address priority problems
- tailor the care plan to meet the specific needs of clients
- establish measurable outcomes
- communicate and coordinate the delivery of care to the clients
- conduct periodic evaluations to ascertain the need for revision
- provide continuity of care

■ **Stroke Client: A Nursing Care Plan. Functional Health Patterns Are the Assessment Framework.**

ASSESSMENT	NURSING DIAGNOSTIC STATEMENT	OUTCOMES	NURSING INTERVENTIONS	CRITICAL THINKING
Subjective Data "I am too weak to walk." "I feel fatigued," "I feel short of breath."	Activity intolerance related to immobility as evidenced by verbalizations of fatigue, inability to walk 5 ft, pulse 100 on exertion	1: Client will demonstrate use of walker accurately by 9/10/97.	Outcome Criterion 1 Date: 9/3/97 Teach client use of walker by 9/8/97. Jolene Vezzetti, RN	Standing and walking extend the knee and hip joints; increases independence.
		2: Daughter will describe plan for home care realistically by 9/20/97.	Outcome Criterion 2 Date: 9/3/97 Refer daughter to visiting nurse by 9/10/97 Jolene Vezzetti, RN	Mutually agreed-upon goal among client, family, and nurse facilitates resolution of client's problems.
Objective Data Unable to walk 5 ft. Pulse 100 on exertion Respirations 28, labored		3: Family friend will walk client 50 feet every evening by 9/30/97.	Outcome Criterion 3 Date: 9/5/97 Instruct family friend of therapeutic effects of ambulation. Jolene Vezzetti, RN	Stress of the weight-bearing on bones decreases calcium loss from bones.
Dysfunctional Health Pattern Activity- Exercise				

■ **Client with a Congenital Heart Dysfunction: A Nursing Care Plan. Body Systems Are the Assessment Framework.**

ASSESSMENT	NURSING DIAGNOSTIC STATEMENT	OUTCOME CRITERIA	NURSING INTERVENTIONS	CRITICAL THINKING
Subjective Data	Ineffective airway clearance related to decreased energy level as evidenced by rapid, shallow respirations, verbal expressions of difficulty breathing, inability to cough up sputum	1. Client will expectorate lung secretions unassisted by 9/20/97.	Outcome Criterion 1 Date: 9/3/97 Teach client to breathe deeply by 9/4/97. Jolene Vezzetti, RN	Voluntary coughing in conjunction with deep breathing facilitates the movement and expectoration of respiratory tract secretions.
"I cannot breathe."				
"I feel plugged up."				
"I cannot cough."				
Objective Data				
Respirations 30, shallow				
Crackling RLL				
Inability to cough up sputum				
		2. Mother will demonstrate use of exygen equipment accurately by 9/30/97.	Outcome Criterion 2 Date: 9/3/97 Explain to mother therapeutic effects of oxygen therapy by 9/20/97. Jolene Vezzetti, RN	Additional oxygen is indicated for clients who have reduced lung diffusion of oxygen through the respiratory membrane. Teaching the family the therapeutic effects of oxygen and use of the equipment will facilitate the home care of the client.
		3. Parents will demonstrate suctioning of child accurately by 9/10/97.	Outcome Criterion 3 Date: 9/3/97 Demonstrate to family suctioning procedure by 9/5/97. Jolene Vezzetti, RN	Family's fears and anxieties will be reduced with an explanation of procedures. Maintaining a patent airway is a high-priority need.
Dysfunctional System Respiratory				

EXERCISE 5–D: WRITING A NURSING CARE PLAN FOR THE MR. LOPEZ SCENARIO

The purpose of exercise 5–D is to provide the learner with the opportunity to write a nursing care plan for the client, Mr. Lopez, in the scenario in Chapter 3. Fill in the spaces below with the requested information. Refer to previous exercises on Mr. Lopez.

ASSESSMENT
Subjective data

_____
_____
_____

Objective data

_____
_____
_____
_____
_____

NURSING DIAGNOSTIC STATEMENT
1. Nursing diagnostic label

_____
_____

Etiology (related to)

_____
_____

_____

Defining characteristics (as evidenced by)

_____
_____
_____

OUTCOME
1a. Subject: _____

Measurable verb: _____

Outcome: _____

Criterion: _____

Target time: _____

1b. Subject _____

Measurable verb: _____

Outcome: _____

Criterion: _____

Target time: _____

NURSING DIAGNOSTIC STATEMENT (CONT)

2. Nursing diagnostic label

_____

_____

Etiology (related to)

_____

_____

Defining characteristics (as evidenced by)

_____

_____

3. Nursing diagnostic label

_____

_____

Etiology (related to)

_____

_____

OUTCOME (CONT)

2a. Subject: _____

Measurable verb: _____

Outcome: _____

Criterion: _____

Target time: _____

2b. Subject: _____

Measurable verb: _____

Outcome: _____

Criterion: _____

Target time: _____

3. Subject: _____

Measurable verb: _____

Outcome: _____

Criterion: _____

Target time: _____

NURSING INTERVENTIONS

1a. Measurable verb: _____

Subject: _____

Outcome: _____

Criterion: _____

Target time: _____

Signature: _____

1b. Measurable verb: _____

Subject: _____

Outcome: _____

Criterion: _____

Target time: _____

Signature: _____

2a. Measurable verb: _____

Subject: _____

Outcome: _____

Criterion: _____

Target time: _____

Signature: _____

2b. Measurable verb: _____

Subject: _____

Outcome: _____

Criterion: _____

Target time: _____

Signature: _____

REVIEW DATE

(state date)

_____

(state date)

_____

(state date)

_____

(state date)

_____

STATEMENT (CONT)

Defining characteristics (as evidenced by)

_____

_____

_____

_____

4. Nursing diagnostic label

_____

Etiology (related to)

_____

_____

_____

Defining characteristics (as evidenced by)

_____

_____

_____

_____

OUTCOME (CONT)

4a. Subject: _____

Measurable verb: _____

Outcome: _____

Criterion: _____

Target time: _____

4b. Subject: _____

Measurable verb: _____

Outcome: _____

Criterion: _____

Target time: _____

4c. Subject: _____

Measurable verb: _____

Outcome: _____

Criterion: _____

Target time: _____

NURSING INTERVENTIONS (CONT)

3. Measurable verb: _____

Subject: _____

Outcome: _____

Criterion: _____

Target time: _____

Signature: _____

4a. Measurable verb: _____

Subject: _____

Outcome: _____

Criterion: _____

Target time: _____

Signature: _____

4b. Measurable verb: _____

Subject: _____

Outcome: _____

Criterion: _____

Target time: _____

Signature: _____

4c. Measurable verb: _____

Subject: _____

Outcome: _____

Criterion: _____

Target time: _____

Signature: _____

REVIEW DATE

_____
(state date)

_____
(state date)

_____
(state date)

_____
(state date)

✓ **CORRECT RESPONSES**

EXERCISE 5–A: *PRIORITY RANKING OF NURSING DIAGNOSES*

NURSING DIAGNOSES	MASLOW'S NEEDS	RANKING
1. Altered urinary elimination	1. Physiologic	1. High
2. Acute pain	2. Physiologic	2. Medium
3. Urge incontinence	3. Physiologic	3. Medium
4. Knowledge deficit	4. Safety	4. Medium

EXERCISE 5–B: *IDENTIFICATION OF OUTCOMES*

1. Nursing diagnosis: <u>Altered urinary elimination</u>
   Outcome
   Date: <u>9/15/97</u>
   Subject: <u>Client</u>
   Measurable verb: <u>will demonstrate</u>
   Outcome: <u>no frequency of urination</u>
   Criteria: <u>evidenced by straw-colored clear urine; negative urine culture</u>
   Target time: <u>within 3 days of initiating antibiotic therapy and increasing fluid intake to 2000 mL/24 hour</u>
2. Nursing diagnosis: <u>Pain</u>
   Outcome
   Date: <u>9/15/97</u>
   Subject: <u>Client</u>
   Measurable verb: <u>will urinate</u>
   Outcome: <u>without discomfort</u>
   Criteria: <u>evidenced by verbalization of no pain or burning upon urination, and no back pain</u>
   Target time: <u>within 24 hours of treatment</u>
3. Nursing diagnosis: <u>Urge incontinence</u>
   Outcome
   Date: <u>9/15/97</u>
   Subject: <u>Client</u>
   Measurable verb: <u>will verbalize</u>
   Outcome: <u>no urgency to void</u>
   Criteria: <u>as evidenced by voiding in amounts normal for the client</u>
   Target time: <u>within 3 days of initiating treatment</u>
4. Nursing diagnosis: <u>Knowledge deficit (prevention of urinary infection)</u>

Outcome
Date: <u>9/15/97</u>
Subject: <u>Client and family</u>
Measurable verb: <u>will verbalize accurately</u>
Outcome: <u>precautionary measures to prevent or reduce the risk of another urinary tract infection</u>
Criteria: <u>accurately</u>
Target time: <u>at the completion of the present clinic visit, and on the follow-up telephone call from the clinic nurse scheduled within 7 days of clinic visit.</u>

EXERCISE 5–C: *WRITING NURSING INTERVENTIONS*

1. Nursing diagnosis: <u>Altered urinary elimination</u>
   Outcome criteria: <u>Client will demonstrate absence of signs and symptoms of a urinary tract infection as evidenced by negative urine cultures; no complaints of pain, burning, urgency, frequency; straw-colored clear urine within 3 days of initiating antibiotic therapy; and increasing fluid intake to 2000 mL/24 hours.</u>
   a. Nursing intervention
      Date written: <u>9/8/97</u>
      Measurable verb: <u>Monitor</u>
      Subject: <u>client's</u>
      Outcome: <u>voiding pattern; record response to treatment noting the frequency, urgency, characteristics of urine</u>
      Target time: <u>immediately</u>
      Signature: <u>Joan Marshall, RN</u>
   b. Nursing intervention
      Date written: <u>9/8/97</u>
      Measurable verb: <u>Teach</u>
      Subject: <u>client</u>
      Outcome: <u>to drink 2000 mL fluids every day (qd) until clear; drink 1500 mL fluids qd thereafter to prevent reinfection</u>
      Target time: <u>Teach immediately; telephone client within 3 days to confirm compliance with instructions</u>
      Signature: <u>Joan Marshall, RN</u>
2. Nursing diagnosis: <u>Pain</u>
   Outcome criteria: <u>Client will urinate without discomfort evidenced by verbalization of no pain or burning on urination within 24 hours of treatment</u>

a. Nursing intervention
Date written: 9/8/97
Measurable verb: Teach
Subject: client
Outcome: to rate pain on a scale of 0–10
(0 = no pain and 10 = excruciating pain)
Target time: immediately
Signature: Joan Marshall, RN

b. Nursing intervention
Date written: 9/8/97
Measurable verb: Administer
Subject: client's
Outcome: pain medications as ordered
Target time: immediately
Signature: Joan Marshall, RN

c. Nursing intervention
Date written: 9/8/97
Measurable verb: Monitor
Subject: client's
Outcome: response to pain medication
Target time: within 30 minutes of administration; at follow-up telephone call
Signature: Joan Marshall, RN

3. Nursing diagnosis: Urge incontinence
Outcome criteria: Client will verbalize no urgency to void evidenced by no frequency voiding in small amounts within 3 days of initiating treatment

d. Nursing intervention
Date written: 9/8/97
Measurable verb: Teach
Subject: client
Outcome: to void at first urge and at least every 2 to 3 hours during the day, one or two times at night to prevent bladder distention
Target time: immediately; at follow-up clinic visit
Signature: Joan Marshall, RN

4. Nursing diagnosis: Knowledge deficit
Outcome criteria: Client will verbalize precautionary measures to prevent or reduce the risk of another urinary tract infection accurately at the completion of the present clinic visit and on the follow-up telephone call from the clinic nurse

a. Nursing intervention
Date written: 9/8/97
Measurable verb: Teach
Subject: client and family
Outcome: signs and symptoms of infection and to seek health care assistance promptly if reinfection occurs
Target time: at first clinic visit; reinforce teaching by follow-up telephone call completed within 7 days of clinic visit
Signature: Joan Marshall, RN

b. Nursing intervention
Date written: 9/8/97
Measurable verb: Teach
Subject: client
Outcome: to avoid caffeine and alcohol, which irritate the bladder
Target time: immediately; at follow-up telephone call
Signature: Joan Marshall, RN

c. Nursing intervention
Date written: 9/8/97
Measurable verb: Teach
Subject: client
Outcome: action and side effects of the prescribed medication(s)
Target time: immediately; at follow-up telephone call
Signature: Joan Marshall, RN

EXERCISE 5–D: *WRITING A NURSING CARE PLAN FOR THE MR. LOPEZ SCENARIO*

Nursing diagnoses are listed according to priority.

ASSESSMENT	NURSING DIAGNOSTIC STATEMENT	OUTCOME CRITERIA	NURSING INTERVENTIONS	REVIEW DATES
Subjective data				
"For past 2 weeks, I go to bathroom a lot; urgent need to hurry to bathroom; burns." Urine dark-orange color; "drink 3 cups coffee a day; tall glass water at night; pass little urine; skin dry; dizzy when stand up."	1. Altered urinary elimination (nursing diagnostic label) related to urinary tract infection (cause) as evidenced by verbal expressions urgency, burning, small amounts urine; foul-smelling, dark-orange color; decreased fluid intake; positive C & S (defining characteristics)	1. Client will demonstrate a negative urine culture; no frequency; straw-colored clear urine within 3 days of initiating antibiotic therapy, increasing fluid intake 2000 mL 24 hours.	1a. Monitor client's voiding pattern; record response to treatment, note frequency, characteristics urine immediately. 1b. Offer and teach client to drink 2000 mL fluid/d now and at home. Joan Marshall, RN	1a. Follow-up call; next clinic visit. 1b. Follow-up call within 24 hours; next clinic visit.
Objective data				
BP 130/80 lying BF 110/70 standing T 100.4°F P 90 foul-smell urine; dark-amber color, cloudy, thick; skin remained tented; fluid intake 780 mL/24 h; sp gr >1.030; C & S positive *E. coli,* sensitive to ampicillin.	2. Pain (nursing diagnostic label) related to irritation bladder/urethral mucosa (cause) as evidenced by verbal description burning sensation on urination, low back pain (defining characteristics)	2. Client will urinate without discomfort evidenced by verbalization no pain/ burning on urination and no lower back pain, within 24 hours of initiating treatment.	2a. Teach client to rate pain on scale 0–10 immediately. 2b. Administer pain medication, reassess client's response immediately and at follow-up telephone call. Joan Marshall, RN	2a. Follow-up call within 7 days. 2b. Follow-up call within 7 days.
	3. Urge incontinence (nursing diagnostic label) related to unresolved urinary tract infection (cause) as evidenced by verbal description burning sensation on urination; low back pain (defining characteristics)	3. Client will verbalize no urgency to void and will void in amounts normal for the client within 3 days of initiating treatment	3 Teach client to void at first urge; at least q2h to q3h during day, 1–2 during night. Joan Marshall, RN	3. Next clinic visit.

NURSING DIAGNOSTIC STATEMENT	**OUTCOME CRITERIA**	**NURSING INTERVENTIONS**	**REVIEW DATES**
4. Knowledge deficit: prevention urinary tract infection (nursing diagnostic label) related to unfamiliarity with information resources (cause) as evidenced by presence UTI 2 weeks; not seek health care treatment (define characteristics)	4. Client and family will accurately verbalize precautionary measures to prevent or reduce risk of reinfection at clinic visit and on follow-up telephone call within 7-days clinic visit and the next clinic visit.	4a. Teach client and family signs and symptoms of infection; seek health care tx. promptly; discuss at first clinic visit; reinforce teaching at follow-up; call within 7-days clinic visit.	4a. Call within 7 days; check at next clinic visit.
		4b. Teach client to avoid caffeine and alcohol (irritate bladder); discuss immediately; at follow-up telephone call.	4b. Call client within 7 days; check at next clinic visit.
		4c. Teach client action/side effects medication(s); immediately; at follow-up call; next clinic visit.	4c. Call within 7 days; review next clinic visit.

Implementation

Nursing and interdisciplinary interventions help clients meet the identified outcomes. If nursing care plans are incorporated into interdisciplinary plans of care, nurses implement those actions that dwell within the domain of nursing.

■ COMPONENTS OF IMPLEMENTATION

- Independent nursing actions (nurse-prescribed)
- Collaborative nursing actions (physician-prescribed; nurse-practitioner–prescribed; physical-therapist–prescribed)
- Documentation of nursing actions and the client's response to nursing care and the care of the interdisciplinary team

● Independent Nursing Actions

What actions can be implemented by the nurse without physician's order and remain within the scope of nursing practice? Independent nursing actions are performed without a physician's order. They may be called nurse-prescribed interventions (McCloskey & Bulachek, 1992). Independent nursing actions are governed by the American Nurses Association Standards of Clinical Nursing Practice (1991), state nurse practice acts, and the policies and procedures of health care facilities.

■ Stroke Client: Independent Nursing Actions

- Assess and reassess client
- Formulate a nursing care plan
- Listen to client's and family's fears and concerns
- Observe and record client's response to care
- Report to the next shift the client's status
- Delegate tasks to nursing staff to meet client needs
- Demonstrate procedures to the client and family
- Perform full range of motion (ROM) four times daily
- Teach quadriceps setting
- Reposition every 2 hours (q2h)
- Inspect skin for signs of injury or pressure
- Assess client's ability to perform activities of daily living (ADL)

■ **Client with Congenital Heart Dysfunction: Independent Nursing Interventions**

- Assess and reassess client
- Auscultate lungs; report crackling, rubbing, gurgling lung sounds to physician
- Report suspected heart murmurs to physician
- Monitor client's weight
- Administer small, frequent meals
- Observe eating patterns
- Observe for signs and symptoms of respiratory tract infection
- Teach the parents auscultation for lung sounds
- Teach the parents to suction client's lungs
- Teach client and family health promotion strategies, including the need to promptly seek treatment of infections
- Teach the parents to take their child's temperature
- Schedule activities to allow maximum rest
- Assist child to select activities appropriate for condition
- Introduce parents to families who have similarly affected children

EXERCISE 6–A: *IDENTIFICATION OF INDEPENDENT NURSING ACTIONS*

In the spaces provided below, list independent nursing actions appropriate for Mr. Lopez (Chapter 3 scenario).

1. _____

2. _____

3. _____

4. _____

5. _____

6. _____

7. _____

8. _____

Correct responses are on p. 72.

• Collaborative Nursing Actions

Collaborative nursing actions are implemented when the nurse works with other health care team members in making joint decisions about resolving the client's problems. Collaborative nursing actions include carrying out physician-prescribed, nurse-practitioner–prescribed, and physical-therapist–prescribed orders, in addition to following an organization's protocols and policies. Protocols and policies state the medications approved by the medical staff for administration by registered nurses. Protocols and policies may differ among organizations. For example, an organization's protocol for emergency treatment of acute angina may permit registered nurses in the emergency room to administer one nitroglycerine tablet every 5 minutes for three doses without having to obtain a specific order, while another emergency room may not permit registered nurses to administer nitroglycerine without a physician's order.

When physicians write orders, they rely on registered nurses and other health care team members to carry them out correctly. If there is a question regarding an order, that is, if the order is ambiguous, nurses review the organization's policy regarding physician orders in addition to contacting the physician for clarification. Physician's orders are written on physician's order sheets; they are a permanent part of the client's medical record.

Components of a physician's order include:

- date and time the order was written
- action to be taken (administer)
- subject (medication)
- route (oral)
- frequency (q4h)
- reason for order (hip pain)

Health care team members, including faculty and student nurses affiliating with a medical center, read the policies and procedures before the implementation of physicians' orders.

■ Stroke Client: Collaborative Nursing Actions

- Discuss discharge planning with interdisciplinary team
- Discuss client's fears with chaplin
- Confer with physical therapy regarding ROM exercise
- Refer client to occupational therapy
- Administer pain medication as ordered by physician

■ Client with Congenital Heart Dysfunction: Collaborative Nursing Actions

- Collect specimens as ordered by physician
- Consult with community nurse regarding home visit
- Refer client to respiratory therapy
- Confer with physician regarding medications
- Consult with dietitian about diet.

EXERCISE 6–B: *IMPLEMENTING COLLABORATIVE NURSING ACTIONS*

In the spaces below, list the collaborative nursing action implemented by the outpatient clinic nurse for Mr. Lopez (Chapter 3 scenario).

1. _____

2. _____

Correct responses are on p. 72.

• Documentation of Interventions and the Client's Responses

Documentation is the act of authenticating events or activities by maintaining written records. The words *documenting, recording,* and *charting* refer to the process of writing notes on the client's medical record (chart). Documentation remains the vehicle for communication from one professional to another about the status of clients.

Medical Records

To organize the documentation by the health care team, a medical record is compiled for each client upon admission or during the initial visit. Entries written in medical records are made by individuals authorized by the organization's policies. Medical records contain the client's history and physical findings, nursing care plans, interdisciplinary plans of care, clinical pathways, and evidence of actions taken by the health care team, and the client's response to these actions.

Medical records are divided into sections and may vary with each health care facility. For example, the medical record may include the following information:

- the problem list of diagnoses
- physicians' order sheet
- copy of advance directive (document whereby clients state the management of end-of-life decisions) if appropriate
- history and physical examination done by the physician
- assessment forms completed by nurses, dietitians, chaplains, and other interdisciplinary team members
- graphic forms (TPR) and other flow sheets (intake and output)
- progress notes, with members of all disciplines writing consecutive entries
- laboratory reports
- informed consents if surgery or other invasive procedures are planned
- copies of other reports (such as x-ray)
- referrals to community agencies
- personal information regarding the client, such as address and telephone of family member

Health care team members may not have day-to-day contact with each other; therefore, entries written in the medical record are essential communication among disciplines to help ensure continuity of care. The client's record provides evidence of the independent and collaborative **nursing actions** implemented by the nurse, the **client's response to those actions,** and **those of the interdisciplinary team,** and changes in the client's condition.

Authenticating Entries into the Medical Record

All entries written in the medical record are authenticated, that is, they are followed by the signature and title of the writer (Joe Schmidt, MD; Sally Smith, RN). If computerized progress notes and reports are used, the electronic signatures, that is, the access and verification codes to gain entry into the system are the legal signatures of practitioners. The signatures of practitioners with access codes are usually filed in information management departments of a facility. The verification code is known only to the practitioner and protects against unauthorized use of electronic signatures. The nurses' notes and the entries by the other members of the health care team are a permanent part of the client's medical record.

Frequency of Charting

The frequency of charting depends on the client's condition, therapies administered, and policies of a facility. In a hospital, the requirement may be to write nurses' notes and complete reassessment forms at least once per shift. Nurses record the client's progress toward resolving the nursing diagnoses noted on the nursing care plan and the medical diagnoses recorded on the interdisciplinary plan of care. Other health care team members address the client's progress on the progress notes.

In long-term-care facilities, a weekly summary note may be written by the nurse or interdisciplinary team members. In an ambulatory clinic or in community health settings, a nurse's note is written for each encounter with the client in addition to the entries written by interdisciplinary team members.

Legal Aspects of Charting

The client's medical record is a legal document and admissible in court during a malpractice suit. Nurses' notes and notes by the interdisciplinary team provide evidence of the nurse's actions and those of the interdisciplinary team. To determine if a registered nurse functioned reasonably (rationally) and prudently (judiciously), a jury will review and compare the nurse's notes and compare the entries with the *ANA Standards of Clinical Nursing Practice* (1991) and standards of practice and care specific to a health care facility. Maintaining confidentiality of the information in the medical record is the responsibility of the entire health care team (unit clerks, nurses, physicians, social workers). Nurses protect the medical records from view of unauthorized readers such as visitors. The nurse verifies the identification and "need to know" of individuals seeking access to medical records. The nurse's signature at the end of a nurse's note signifies accountability for the contents of the entry. Alteration of a legal document is a felony; it is unacceptable to obliterate the writing on a chart by using white-out, markers, erasers, ink, or other materials, it must be crossed out and initialled (see Guidelines for Accurate Charting, p. 70).

Charting in Military Time or Greenwich Time

Entries in the medical record indicate the time of the entry and the time a procedure or treatment was performed. To increase the accuracy of identifying the times, the Greenwich time system is applied in the majority of health care facilities and the military. Greenwich time uses a 24-hour clock and eliminates confusion about whether a time was AM or PM In military time, a four digit number indicates the hours and minutes. A health care facility's policies will state the correct format for citing time.

COMPARISON OF MILITARY AND GREENWICH TIME

Military Time	Civilian Time
0100	1:00 AM
0200	2:00 AM
0215	2:15 AM
1200	12:00 PM (noon)
1300	1:00 PM
1420	2:20 PM
1800	6:00 PM
0001	12:01 AM (midnight)

■ TYPES OF CHARTING

Health care systems implement various types of documentation formats.

- Preprinted assessment and reassessment forms
- Narrative progress notes
- SOAP charting
- ADPIE and APIE notes
- FOCUS notes
- flow sheets and graphic records
- charting by exception

Each format denotes the subjective and objective data, the nurse's and interdisciplinary team's actions, and the client's response to the actions. Graphic records and flow sheets depict the temperature, pulse, respirations, blood pressure; intake and output; medications administered; and daily nursing care.

● Preprinted Assessment and Reassessment Forms

To facilitate data collection and expedite the assessment step, many facilities use preprinted assessment and reassessment forms that clearly delineate the data

necessary for collection. With fewer health care workers (nurses), subjective and objective data collection may be expedited. Preprinted assessment forms provide clues to remind nurses of information required. Facilities may use structured forms within a framework (functional health patterns; body systems). There is a trend to use preprinted interdisciplinary assessment forms to coordinate and eliminate having various members of the health care team collect the same information. Nurses should avoid rewriting the information documented on a preprinted assessment form in the body of the nurses' notes unless there is a need to elaborate a finding.

Advantages of Preprinted Assessment Forms. In facilities with fewer licensed health care providers and growing numbers of nonprofessional providers, preprinted assessment forms organize and expedite the collection of data. Bedside computers, computers available in the outpatient clinics, and laptop computers for community nurses facilitate the entry of data at the point of care. Using computers to record care permits rapid retrieval of data.

Disadvantages of Preprinted Assessment Forms. The disadvantage of preprinted assessment forms is that nurses and other health care providers assess only the information listed on the form and fail to assess other responses of the clients. Another disadvantage of computerized forms is that the breakdown or shutdown of the computer system temporarily makes the information unavailable.

Following is part of an admission assessment form for Gordon's 11 Functional Health Patterns as the format (see Chapter 8 for additional information on assessment of functional health patterns).

ELIMINATION PATTERN

Subjective Data	Objective Data
History:	
Nausea _____	Abdomen
Vomiting _____	Soft _____ Firm _____
Dysphagia _____	Nontender _____ Tender _____
No problem _____	Nondistended _____
Bowel Habits:	Distended _____
Stools per day _____	Bowel sounds _____
Soft/formed _____	Bowel sounds absent _____
Constipation _____	Ostomies _____ Type _____
Diarrhea _____	Tubes _____ Type _____
Incontinence _____	

● Narrative Progress Notes

Narrative charting is a description of information about the clients. The information is recorded chronologically. In some agencies separate columns are provided to chart treatments, nursing diagnoses and medical diagnoses, and the observations regarding the client's response to care. Begin the narrative note with the nursing diagnosis or medical diagnosis, state the subjective and objective data, interventions implemented, and the client's responses to care.

Advantages of Narrative Charting.
The advantages to narrative charting include:

- charting is ongoing throughout the shift
- events are written in order of their occurrence
- notes describe subjective and objective data, nursing actions, and the client's response to nursing actions
- notes are written in brief, concise phrases, not complete sentences
- notes may be interspersed between SOAP, FOCUS, ADPIE entries

Disadvantages of Narrative Charting.
One disadvantage of narrative charting is the difficulty encountered in finding data about a specific problem without examining all of the recorded information. For this reason, flow sheets and graphic records are helpful in measuring specific variables. In addition, narrative notes are more time-consuming to write than other charting formats.

NARRATIVE NOTE
9/3/97   Nurse's note: High Risk for Infection
2200   "My arm is burning." IV running left forearm. Left forearm erythematous, edematous, warm, painful to touch. IV discontinued. Warm soaks applied. Temperature 100° F. orally Physician notified. IV nurse notified to restart IV another site. Beatrice Ryan, RN.

• SOAP Charting

SOAP charting is employed with Problem Oriented Medical Records (POMR), which reflects the problems identified by members of the health care team. The problems are listed in front of the client's chart in chronologic order, according to the date on which each problem was identified. In managing clients' care, the health care team records SOAP charting on the progress notes. The charting portrays a continuous picture of the client's progress toward resolution of the problems.

Components of Soap Charting.
SOAP charting consists of four parts:

- **S**ubjective data
- **O**bjective data

- Analysis of the data (What does the information mean?)
- **P**lan for resolving the problem

The acronyms SOAPIE and SOAPIER refer to formats that add implementation (**I**), evaluation (**E**), and revision (**R**) to the documentation. Many health care practitioners use only the SOAP format.

S:	**Subjective**	In quotation marks, the nurse writes the exact comments of the client.
O:	**Objective**	The nurse records the data that nurse saw, heard, smelled, or touched.
A:	**Analysis**	What does the data mean? The nurse analyzes (examines) and interprets the meaning of the subjective and objective data. Progress toward resolving the nursing diagnoses is noted ("Ineffective airway clear remains unresolved"). The analysis reflects the nurse's critical thinking and clinical judgment.
P:	**Plan**	The nurse records the plan to resolve the problem identified in the analysis.

Advantages of SOAP Charting.
The nurse correlates SOAP charting with the nursing diagnoses noted on the nursing care plan and the medical diagnoses listed on the problem list. The nurse records the client's progress toward resolution of the problems.

Disadvantage of SOAP Charting.
The SOAP note fails to show the sequence of events.

PROGRESS NOTE USING SOAP CHARTING
9/4/97   *Physician's Note: Diabetes mellitus*
0900   S: "I eat a lot of candy bars and cokes."
          O: 9/2/97 FBS 250. Ht. 5'8'. Wt. 205 lb.
          A: Uncontrolled diabetes.
          P: Referral to dietitian. Consult with diabetes clinical nurse specialist regarding instruction on insulin administration and foot care. Order insulin coverage.————————John Smith, MD

9/4/97   *Nurse's Note: Noncompliance with thera-*
1100   *peutic regimen.*
          S: "I stopped giving myself insulin. You are the nurse. You give it to me."
          O: Drew up insulin incorrectly. Refused to give self insulin injection. Threw syringe on floor.

A: Noncompliance with therapeutic regimen continues.

P: Discuss therapeutic effects insulin with client and wife. Client will reiterate instructions. Return insulin demonstration 10/1/97 at 0700. Discussed attending diabetic classes at 1400, 10/1/97 with client and wife.—Jane Green, RN

9/4/97 *Dietitian's Note: Diabetes mellitus*
1200 S: "I eat mostly vegetables, fruit."

O: Ate 50% food on lunch tray. Ate 1 medium apple and carrots. Cottage cheese, milk, wheat bread not consumed. Unable verbalize allowable foods on American Diabetes Association (ADA) exchange list.

A: Knowledge deficit of prescribed diet.

P: Attend diabetic class on diabetic diets, 9/5/97 at 1400. Client will write diet diary.——————Mary Smith, RD

9/5/97 *Social Worker's Note: Home Care*
0900 S: "My wife does not cook the food on my diet. She says it is too much trouble."

O: Wife failed to keep scheduled appointment today with client and social worker.

A: High risk for ineffective coping by wife.

P: Call wife today. Assess concerns. Reschedule appointment for this week.—Mary Brown, Social Worker

---

■ **Stroke Client: SOAP Charting**

9/7/97 0900 *Physician's Note: Cerebrovascular Accident (CVA)*

S: "I feel congested. My chest hurts when I take a deep breath."

O: Crackling sounds RLL. Chest x-ray reveals right lower lobe infiltration. Sputum positive for streptococcus pneumonia.

A: Pneumonia due to immobility; decreased lung expansion.

P: Treat with (IVP) antibiotics based on sensitivity results.————
Brenda Bullen, MD

9/7/97 1000 *Nurses's Note: Ineffective Airway Clearance*

S: "I'm short of breath. I told the Dr. that it hurts to breathe."

O: Respirations 26, shallow, Crackling RLL.

A: Decreased lung expansion due to immobility. Ineffective airway clearance persists.

P: Teach client to splint chest when coughing. Provide humidifier. Increase fluid intake to 2000 mL qd. Consult with Dr. regarding chest physiotherapy.————
Jolene Vezzetti, RN

9/7/97 1200 Dietitian's Note: Special Diet.

S: "I can't eat now. I'm too tired."

O: Consumed 25% lunch; consumed liquids only.

A: Decreased energy level limits ability to eat solid food; alteration in nutrition, less than body requirements prevails.

P: Offer liquid blenderized diet during acute phase pneumonia. Daily intake 1500 calories. Progress to small frequent feedings.————
Steve Byrum, RD

● **Modified SOAP Charting**

Modified SOAP charting may be entered by licensed practical nurses and nursing assistants according to the health care facility's policy.

COMPONENTS OF MODIFIED SOAP CHARTING

S: **Subjective** In quotation marks, record the exact comments of the client.

O: **Objective** Record the data that is seen, heard, smelled, or felt. The objective data validates the subjective data.

AT: **Action** Actions the licensed practical nurse or nursing assistant implements to resolve the problem noted in the subjective and objective data.

■ **Client with Congenital Heart Dysfunction:**
Nurse's Note by Licensed Practical Nurse
or Nursing Assistant

9/3/97   Nurse's Note
1300   S: "I feel dizzy."
       O: BP 90/50. Unsteady gait. Diaph-
           oretic.
     AT: Assisted to bed. Charge nurse in-
           formed.————Susan Deer, LPN

• **ADPIE and APIE Charting**

ADPIE and APIE are documentation forms similar to SOAP. The ADPIE format follows:

A:	**Assessment**	Combines the subjective and objective data. Subjective data are written in quotation marks.
D:	**Diagnoses**	Nursing or medical diagnoses are listed.
P:	**Plan**	Includes proposed nursing and interdisciplinary interventions and client's outcomes.
I:	**Implementation**	Enters the nursing and interdisciplinary interventions noted on the care plan that were actually fulfilled for the clients.
E:	**Evaluation**	Consists of the response of the clients to nursing and interdisciplinary interventions and the attainment of identified outcomes.

APIE is a similar format of charting that condenses the client's data into fewer statements: **A**ssessment, **P**lan, **I**mplementation, and **E**valuation.

• **FOCUS Charting**

In Focus charting, the nurses note focus or concentrate on specific problems and concerns and like SOAP charting, key words are used to organize the written entries.

Components of FOCUS.   FOCUS charting consists of the Focus statement, **D**ata statement, **A**ction statement, **R**esponse of the client statement, and **T**eaching statement (DART).

FOCUS:	The Focus statement is the nursing diagnosis or a concern regarding the client, client's behavior (inability to recall directions, for exam-

ple), acute changes in the client's status (such as amputation of a leg), and pivotal events (for example, falls) in the client's therapy that influence previously identified outcomes.

DATA:	The nurse notes the subjective and objective data that support the nursing diagnosis or medical diagnosis.
ACTION:	Actions reflect the immediate or future nursing and interdisciplinary team's actions to resolve the problems or concerns.
RESPONSE:	The nurse and interdisciplinary team describe the client's response to the interventions.
TEACHING:	The nurse and the interdisciplinary team describe the teaching to assist the client in resolving the problem.

■ **Client with Congenital Heart Dysfunction:**
Focus Charting

9/7/97   Nurse's Note Focus: Ineffective airway
        clearance
1100   DATA: "I am short of breath. I told the Dr. that my chest hurts when I breathe."
        Rated pain 6 on scale 0–10. R 30, shallow. Crackling sounds RLL. Inability to cough up sputum.
1110   ACTION: Physician called. Nasal suctioning,expectorant, inhalation therapy, room humidifier ordered.
1130   Respiratory therapist (RT) administered inhalation therapy. RT stated suctioning not required. Humidifier in room. Expectorant administered.
1135   RESPONSE: Expectorated moderate amount tenacious yellow sputum unassisted.
1200   TEACHING: Taught to deep breathe and cough following inhalation therapy for 5 minutes every hour to clear lungs. Increase fluid intake to 1500 mL qd. Taught inform nurse before pain rating reaches 4.————————Sarah Duff, RN

Advantages of Focus Charting.   Focus charting facilitates the documentation of nursing and medical diagnoses and compels nurses and the interdisciplinary team to organize their thoughts succinctly. The DART format provides a complete, concise description of each focus of care.

Disadvantage of Focus Charting.   Focus charting fails to show the sequence of events.

• Flow Sheets and Graphic Records

Flow sheets and graphic forms reflect the client variables that are frequently monitored by nurses and the interdisciplinary team.

Advantages of Flow Sheets and Graphic Records.   Specific variables such as temperature, pulse, respiration, blood pressure, medications, intake and output are easily recorded on a flow sheet, graphic record, or computerized program. A flow sheet or graphic record reduces the amount of narrative writing by nurses and the interdisciplinary team. The time parameters for flow sheets and graphic records vary from minutes to days. For example, in a critical care unit, the blood pressure is monitored frequently, whereas in community health, the vital signs may be monitored once a month. Abnormal data on the flow sheets and graphic records may be elaborated in the nurses' notes with additional relevant details.

Disadvantages of Flow Sheets and Graphic Records. Failure to elaborate on the progress notes the changes observed in client's condition leads to an incomplete record.

• Charting by Exception

Charting by exception is a documentation system in which only significant (important) findings, exceptions, deviations, or variances to established standards and norms are recorded. Minimum criteria for client care are identified by the *ANA Standards of Clinical Nursing Practice* (1991). In addition, organizations may use unit-based standards of clinical practice, approved protocols, and interdisciplinary clinical pathways to identify the minimum criteria for client care. There may be use of unique flow sheets that specify data required during the assessment and reassessment step and the norms for the data.

Advantages of Charting by Exception.   Charting by exception saves time and eliminates repetitive charting. For example, when a clinical pathway is used, it is expected that the client will travel along the path and meet the outcomes. If the client demonstrates deviations along the pathway, nurses and interdisciplinary team members chart these variances.

Disadvantages of Charting by Exception.   If nurses or other health care professionals fail to chart a variance, it is assumed the outcomes were met.

■ WRITING LEGALLY SOUND NURSES' NOTES

When writing nurses' notes, "think jury"; that is, what type of picture did the notes convey about the nurse's actions toward the client? Nurses' notes transmit facts about the clients and staff delivering the care. To facilitate the writing of legally sound notes, avoid conveying **judgmental opinions** and inferences by interpreting the client's comments in the nurse's own words or imposing the nurse's personal viewpoint. Words such as *seems* and *appears,* which leave room for inferences, are not measurable and may convey an incorrect meaning.

What constitutes inference and fact charting?

Inference:	Poor appetite. What is considered a poor appetite? The word poor is not measurable.
Fact:	Client ate 10% breakfast food: 120 mL coffee, 1 piece wheat toast.

(The amounts are quantified and measurable. The reader of the nurse's notes will know the client's exact intake for breakfast.)

Inference:	Client appears restless.
Fact:	"I did not sleep last night. I feel uptight about my daughter's problems." Pacing floor during interview. Wringing hands. Smoked 10 cigarettes in 20 minute period.

The nurse's note stated the facts, that is, the comments heard (subjective data) and behaviors observed (objective data).

Words That Reflect Inferences.
Avoid Using in Charting

alert	fair
ambulating well	good
anxious	great
apparently	improving
appears	inadvertently
assume	incompetent
combative	"I feel . . ."
conclude	inferior
confused	irritable
coping well	"I think . . ."
depressed	large
difficult	little
disruptive	managing well
doing well	mild withdrawal
eating well	much
emotionally unstable	nervous

obnoxious	slight
poor	uncooperative
refused to cooperate	unexplainable
restless	unfortunately
rude	unstable
seems	well

■ COMPUTER CHARTING

Computers facilitate recording client data. In addition, the quality of care is enhanced when nurses are relieved of clerical duties and charting information is readily available. Computers may be located at the client's bedside in a medical center and in a examining room in an outpatient clinic. Many facilities are targeting the year 2000 for producing totally computerized medical records. In this system of charting, a nurse receives a computer code that is considered the nurse's legal signature.

■ GUIDELINES FOR ACCURATE CHARTING

- Identify the client's name on the chart or computer record prior to writing or entering notes.
- Stamp client's name and identification number on each page in chart.
- Write legibly; print if your writing is difficult to read.
- Type accurately for computer entries.
- Write in black ink.
- All entries begin with the time and date. In the body of the note, state the date and time of the event being described if it differs from the entry time and date.
- End notes with legal signature, first and last name and abbreviated title (RN). Print and sign your name if your signature is not legible.
- Organize entries to flow in logical order of events.
- Chart on a timely basis, that is, as events occur.
- Avoid writing abbreviations; a jury will not understand their meaning (SOB: shortness of breath).

- Records are chronologic. Write on consecutive lines and pages. Avoid leaving blanks in lines of writing. Draw a single line to end of the line to fill the blank space.
- Avoid leaving blank lines between entries; draw a line through a blank that is between entries.
- Print a large *X* to fill rest of blank page that contains no writing.
- If a writing error occurs, draw a single line through the word(s) and initial above it; do not obliterate the word or words. Follow facility instructions for correcting an error on computerized records.
- Do not use white-out to correct errors on the nurses' notes or other records; do not erase errors. Alteration of a legal document is a felony.
- Do not write in margins or squeeze entries between lines.
- Recopy a damaged page of the record onto another page, exactly as written. Do not destroy the original; the original page remains part of the permanent chart. Cross-reference the two pages. On the copy write, *Recopied from page 000* and on the original write, *Recopied on page 000.*
- In charting late entries, write the date and time the late entry is written. In the body of the note, record the date and time the action occurred, the late note, signature and title.
- Document noncompliant behavior; for example, "I will not attend group therapy today."
- A capital letter begins each thought. A period completes each thought; for example, Dyspneic upon exertion. Ate 25% breakfast food.
- Omit the word *client,* as the medical record belongs to the client.
- Spell words correctly.
- Document precise measurements (metric) to ensure accuracy (Drank 200 mL water).
- It is illegal to remove and destroy pages from the medical records.

EXERCISE 6-C: *WRITING A NURSE'S NOTE*

Write a nurse's note based on the scenario of Mr. Lopez in Chapter 3. The student may write notes in the narrative, SOAP, or FOCUS formats using the nursing diagnoses identified in exercise 5–D.

A NARRATIVE NURSE'S NOTE

DATE	TIME	NURSING DIAGNOSIS

A SOAP NURSE'S NOTE

DATE	TIME	NURSING DIAGNOSIS

S:

O:

A:

P:

FOCUS NURSE'S NOTE

DATE	TIME	NURSING DIAGNOSIS

D:

A:

R:

T:

Correct responses on p. 73.

 CORRECT RESPONSES

EXERCISE 6–A: *IDENTIFYING INDEPENDENT NURSING ACTIONS*

1. Monitor client's voiding pattern; teach client to record response to treatment (tx) noting the frequency of urination, urgency, characteristics of urine daily.
2. Teach client to drink 2000 mL fluid qd until urine clears; drink 1500 mL qd to prevent reinfection; teach immediately; telephone client within 3 days to confirm compliance with instructions.
3. Teach the client to rate pain on a scale of 0–10 (0 = no pain and 10 = excruciating pain) immediately.
4. Monitor client's response to pain medication within 30 minutes of administration; at follow-up telephone call.
5. Teach client to void at first urge and at least every 2 to 3 hours (q2–3h) during the day; one or two times at night to prevent bladder distention; immediately; at follow-up clinic visit.
6. Teach client and family signs and symptoms of infection and to seek health care assistance promptly if reinfection occurs, at first clinic visit; reinforce teaching by follow-up telephone call completed within 7 days of clinic visit.
7. Teach client to avoid caffeine and alcohol, which irritate the bladder, immediately; at follow-up telephone call.
8. Teach client the action and side effects of the prescribed medication(s) immediately; reinforce at follow-up telephone call.

EXERCISE 6–B: *IMPLEMENTING COLLABORATIVE NURSING ACTIONS*

1. Administer client's pain medication immediately.
2. Obtain a urine specimen for culture and sensitivity.

EXERCISE 6–C: *WRITING A NURSE'S NOTE*

NARRATIVE FORMAT

09/30/97 1300 Nursing diagnosis: Altered urinary elimination

Arrived in clinic c/o "For the past 2 weeks, I have had to go to the bathroom a lot, and I only pass a little urine . . .I feel a need to hurry to the bathroom. It burns when I pass my water, it smells strong and is dark orange . . .I drink 3 cups coffee day and a tall glass water at night . . .my skin feels dry . . .I get dizzy when I stand up . . .my lower back hurts." In no acute distress. TPR 100.4F; P 90; BP lying 130/80; BP standing 110/70. Urine C & S obtained; foul-smelling, dark amber color, cloudy, thick. Fluid intake past 24 hours 780 mL, sp gr >1.030. Taught to drink 2000 mL fluid/24 hours qd. Interpreter utilized to include wife in teaching. Joan Marshall, RN

SOAP FORMAT

09/30/97 Nursing diagnosis: Pain

S: "For past 2 weeks I go to bathroom a lot . . .pass a little urine . . .I feel a need to hurry to the bathroom . . .it burns when I pass my water. It smells strong and is dark orange . . .I drink 3 cups coffee day and tall glass water at night . . .my skin feels dry . . .I get dizzy when I stand up . . .my lower back hurts"

O: T 100.4F, P 90, BP lying 130/80; BP standing 110/70. Urine foul-smelling, dark amber, cloudy, thick. Intake pst 24 hours 780cc, sp gr >1.030. C & S sent to lab.

A: Acute pain related to urinary tract infection

P: Teach client drink 2000 mL/qd until urine clear; drink 1500 mL/qd prevent recurrence; interpreter utilized to include wife in teaching. Joan Marshall, RN

FOCUS FORMAT

09/30/97 1300 Focus: Knowledge deficit

D: "For past 2 weeks, I go to bathroom a lot . . .only pass little urine . . .I feel a need to hurry to the bathroom . . . burns when I pass my water, it smells strong, dark orange; I drink 3 cups coffee day and tall glass water at night . . .my skin feels dry . . .dizzy when I stand up . . .my lower back hurts." T 100.4F, P 90, BP lying 130/80, BP standing 110/70. Urine foul-smelling, dark amber, cloudy, thick, sp gr >1.030. Intake 780 mL past 24 hours.

A: C & S sent to lab. Telephone advice nurse's number given client and wife for guidance regarding medical problems arising in future.

R: Client and wife stated, "We realize the importance of seeking medical care before he gets into trouble."

T: Taught drink 2000 mL qd until urine clear; then drink 1500 mL qd prevent reinfection. Interpreter utilized to include wife in teaching. Joan Marshall, RN

Evaluation of Outcomes

In the evaluation step of the problem-solving process, observed results are compared with outcomes established during planning. Clients exit the problem-solving process cycle when the outcomes have been achieved; they reenter the cycle if the outcomes were not met (Fig. 7–1).

■ COMPONENTS OF EVALUATION

- Achievement of outcomes
- Effectiveness of the problem-solving approach
- Revision or termination of the nursing care plan, interdisciplinary plan of care, or clinical pathway

• Achievement of Outcomes

What evidence supports achievement of the outcomes? How realistic were the outcomes? As previously discussed, clinical practice guidelines (Agency for Health Care Policy and Research [AHCPR] guidelines) identify outcomes for the care of typical clients (stroke clients) in typical situations and may aid nurses and interdisciplinary teams in evaluating care. Setting a target date for achievement of outcomes also provides a yardstick for measurement. Prior to discharge from a hospital, a discharge planner or an interdisciplinary team may meet to review the plan of care and clinical pathways previously developed for the client and evaluate if the team contributed to the resolution of identified problems. Documentation by the interdisciplinary team provides evidence that outcomes were met (client administered insulin correctly). When they are achieved, the word *resolved* and the date are written on the nursing care plans, interdisciplinary plans of care, and clinical pathways. If the outcomes were not met (client failed to administer insulin correctly), nurses and the interdisciplinary team reassess the client and revise the plans and pathways. Whether the client is in the hospital or cared for in an outpatient facility, if a team fails to evaluate the plan or clinical pathway at regularly scheduled times, the client's outcomes may not be met in a systematic manner. To prevent this problem, a case manager may be assigned to a client to facilitate the delivery of care and the attainment of identified outcomes.

■ **Stroke Client: Achievement of Outcome Confirmed by Comments in Nurses' Note**

Outcome: Daughter will describe plan for client's care at home realistically by 9/30/97.

9/30/97 Nurse's note: Activity intolerance
  S: Daughter stated, "I plan to hire a nurse's aide to care for my father during the day, while I am at work."
  O: Social worker's note confirms nurse's aide has been hired.
  A: Activity intolerance persists.
  P: Community nurse will teach nurse's aide to perform range of motion (ROM) to client's extremities qid.

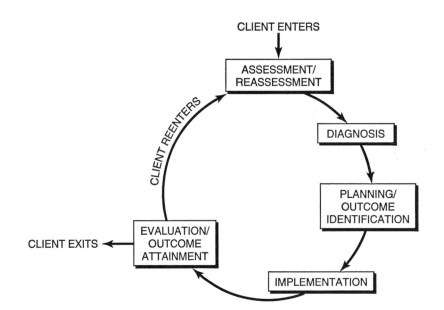

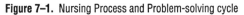

CLIENT ENTERS

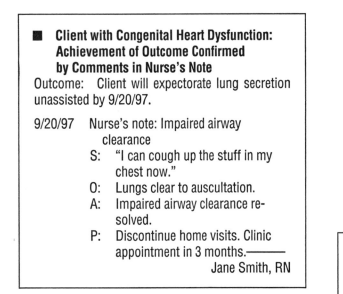

Figure 7–1. Nursing Process and Problem-solving cycle

■ **Client with Congenital Heart Dysfunction: Achievement of Outcome Confirmed by Comments in Nurse's Note**

Outcome: Client will expectorate lung secretion unassisted by 9/20/97.

9/20/97   Nurse's note: Impaired airway clearance
   S: "I can cough up the stuff in my chest now."
   O: Lungs clear to auscultation.
   A: Impaired airway clearance re-solved.
   P: Discontinue home visits. Clinic appointment in 3 months.———
                                    Jane Smith, RN

• **Effectiveness of the Problem-solving Process**

How accurate were the steps of the problem-solving process? What factors hindered achievement of the outcome? Factors affecting the achievement of outcomes may oc-cur throughout the problem-solving process. For example, progress may be impeded by the following:

  • information gaps occurring in the assessment and reassessment (Step 1)

  • wrong nursing or medical diagnosis identified (Step 2)
  • nursing and interdisciplinary interventions not congruent with outcome criteria (Step 3)
  • failure to implement the nursing care plan, interdisciplinary plan of care, or clinical pathway (Step 4)
  • failure to evaluate the client's progress (Step 5)
  • failure of the interdisciplinary team to coordinate efforts to help the client achieve outcomes (All steps)

■ **Stroke Client: Failure to Achieve Outcome Confirmed by the Nurse's Note**

Outcome: Family friend will walk client 50 feet every evening by 9/30/97.

9/30/97   Nurses note: Activity intolerance
1300   Family friend out of town on business for month of September. Client un-able to walk 10 feet unassisted. Wife unable to walk client. Outcome criteria not met. Confer with wife and social worker regarding home care assistance by 10/1/97.———
                                    Sally Smith, RN

■ **Client with Congenital Heart Dysfunction: Failure to Achieve Outcome Confirmed by the Nurse's Note**

Outcome: Mother will demonstrate use of oxygen equipment accurately by 9/30/97.

9/25/97 Nurses note: Ineffective airway clearance. Mother states, "I am afraid to use the oxygen tank." Nurse re-demonstrated use of oxygen tank. Mother refused to return demonstration. Repeat demonstration tomorrow. Outcome criteria not met. Refer to visiting nurse upon discharge.
————————Katherine Bradley, RN.

• **Revision or Termination of the Nursing Care Plan, Interdisciplinary Plan of Care, or Clinical Pathway**

Is the client ready to exit the problem solving cycle? What revisions are required in the plans or clinical pathways? With the achievement of outcomes, the client exits the problem-solving process, and the plans or clinical pathways are terminated. Nurses and inter-disciplinary team members write a discharge note summarizing resolution of nursing and medical diagnoses. The discharge notes indicate the client's status on release from the health care system. Vital signs, procedures taught, medications, self-care abilities, support system, and follow-up appointments are examples of information included in a discharge note.

If the outcomes were not met, the client reenters the problem solving cycle. Nurses and the interdisciplinary team reassess the client and revise the nursing care plan, interdisciplinary plan of care, or clinical pathways to meet continuing needs. A referral to other health care workers in the community may be written to provide continuity of care. For example, a referral to a home health nurse may be written, requesting that the nurse observe the client administering insulin at home.

■ **Stroke Client: Discharge Note**

9/30/97 Nurse's Discharge Summary
1100 Nursing diagnosis: Activity intolerance Walked 50 feet in hallway with walker. Family friend attended physical therapy session with client 9/29/97. Family friend verbalized therapeutic effects of ambulation. Daughter demonstrated ROM all joints correctly. Daughter identified plan for home care. Outcome met. ————————John Kemp, RN

■ **Client with Congenital Heart Dysfunction: Discharge Note**

9/30/97 Nurses Discharge Summary
1400 Nursing diagnosis: Impaired airway clearance. Mother administered oxygen therapy correctly. Client expectorates own secretions. Lungs clear to auscultation. Outcome met. Home visit by visiting nurse 10/1/97.————
Sally Craig, RN

EXERCISE 7–A: *EVALUATION OF THE ACHIEVEMENT OF OUTCOMES*

In this exercise evaluate whether the outcomes noted on the nursing care plan for Mr. Lopez, Exercise 5–D have been met. Write an evaluation of whether the outcomes listed in Exercise 5–D were met based on the continuation of the Lopez scenario below.

Mr. Lopez Scenario, continued

On 10/14/97, Mr. Lopez returned for his scheduled clinic visit. He appeared in no acute distress. He stated that "I no longer have an urgent need to pass my water, and it does not burn anymore. The pain in my lower back is gone." Mr. Lopez stated that the clinic nurse called him about a week after his last visit to check if he was taking his antibiotics and drinking fluids. He said that he "drank about 10 glasses of water or juice a day and now drinks around 7 to 8 large glasses of water or juice a day." Mr. Lopez stated, "I now know that when I first start to have a burning sensation when I pass my water, I need to get help right away." A urine culture was negative. The urine appeared clear, straw-colored, and with no foul odor. Mr. Lopez's blood pressure lying was 140/80, and standing blood pressure was 136/80; pulse 75; and temperature orally 98.6°F. When the nurse pinched Mr. Lopez's skin and released it, the skin immediately sprang back to its normal position.

1. Outcome: Client will demonstrate a negative urine culture; no urgency, no frequency of urination; straw-colored clear urine within 3 days of initiating the antibiotic therapy; increasing fluid intake 2000 mL per 24 hours until urine clear; 1500 mL daily thereafter.
   Resolved: YES _____   NO _____
   Evaluation: _____
   _____
   _____
   _____
   _____
   _____
   _____

2. Outcome: Client will urinate without discomfort evidenced by verbalization of no pain or burning upon urination, and no lower-back pain within 24 hours of initiating treatment.
   Resolved: YES _____   NO _____
   Evaluation: _____
   _____
   _____
   _____
   _____
   _____
   _____

3. Outcome: Client will verbalize no urgency to void, and will void in amounts normal for the client within 3 days of initiating treatment.
   Resolved: YES ____   NO ____
   Evaluation: _____

   _____
   _____
   _____
   _____
   _____
   _____

4. Outcome: Client and family will accurately verbalize precautionary measures to prevent or reduce the risk of reinfection on at the follow-up telephone call within 7-days of the initial clinic visit, and at the next clinic visit.
   Resolved: YES ____   NO ____
   Evaluation: _____

   _____
   _____
   _____
   _____
   _____
   _____
   _____

✔ **CORRECT RESPONSES**

EXERCISE 7-A: EVALUATION OF THE ACHIEVEMENT OF OUTCOME

1. Outcome: Client will demonstrate a negative urine culture; no frequency of urination; straw-colored clear urine within 3 days of initiating the antibiotic therapy; increased fluid intake 2000 mL per 24-hours until urine clear; 1500 mL daily thereafter.
   Resolved: YES _X_   NO ____
   Evaluation: Client verbalized no frequency of urination. Urine culture negative after taking the antibiotics for 3 days. Nurse observed urine specimen was clear, straw-colored, and with no foul odor. Client verbalized that he drank 10 glasses of water (200 ml) per 24 hours until urine was clear, and now drinks 7 to 8 glasses of water every 24 hours.

2. Outcome: Client will urinate without discomfort evidenced by verbalization of no pain or burning upon urination, and no lower-back pain within 24 hours of initiating treatment.
   Resolved: YES _X_   NO ____

   Evaluation: Client verbalized no burning upon urination and no back pain after 24 hours of initiating antibiotics and increasing fluid intake.

3. Outcome: Client will verbalize no urgency to void, and will void in amounts normal for the client within 3 days of initiating treatment.
   Resolved: YES _X_   NO ____
   Evaluation: Client verbalized no urgency to void, and voided in amounts normal for him within 3 days of initiating treatment.

4. Outcome: Client and family will accurately verbalize precautionary measures to prevent or reduce the risk of reinfection the follow-up telephone call within 7-days of the initial clinic visit, and at the next clinic visit.
   Resolved: YES _X_   NO ____
   Evaluation: Client and wife (through an interpreter) verbalized precautionary measures to prevent or reduce the risk of reinfection at follow-up clinic visit. Client stated he reduced the amount of coffee he drank to one cup at breakfast.

Case Study Using Functional Health Patterns

In the case study in this chapter, the nurse focuses on the client's responses to a medical problem. The study is presented in the assessment framework of a nursing model, Gordon's 11 Functional Health Patterns. The model represents sequences of behavior, that is, ways of living (Gordon, 1989). Nursing models facilitate identifying human responses to problems and guide the nurse in selecting appropriate nursing diagnoses. In this chapter, functional health patterns denote the assessment framework for a medical case study: Mr. James Hill is a client with rheumatoid arthritis. The case studies presented in this chapter and Chapter 9 facilitate use of this book throughout the curriculum and in health care facilities.

Following are clustered subjective and objective data related to each functional health pattern. The lists are not inclusive.

■ PATTERN 1: HEALTH PERCEPTION AND HEALTH MANAGEMENT

Describes the client's perception and management of health and well-being.

Subjective Data
Medical and social history
Expectation of health care
Ongoing treatment unrelated to admission diagnosis
Client's perception of health status and well-being
Effect of cultural values on health practices
Activities initiated to keep healthy life-style (jogging)
History of accidents and falls
Absences from school or work
Smoking, drinking, use of illicit drugs

Objective Data
White blood cell count
Ability to set goals
Knowledge of health practices
Hygiene, grooming
Age
Occupational hazards
Record of immunizations

■ PATTERN 2: NUTRITIONAL AND METABOLIC

Describes dietary intake; fluid and electrolyte balance; condition of skin, hair, nails, and teeth; breast-feeding and infant feeding patterns.

Subjective Data
Problems eating, swallowing, digesting
Nausea
Use of alcohol
Routine hair, skin, nail, and mouth care
Allergies to food
Urticaria
Weight changes
Food preferences
Appetite
Family pattern of eating
Influence of culture on diet

Objective Data
Ability to swallow
Nasogastric tube
Daily caloric intake
Intravenous fluids

Total parenteral nutrition (TPN)
Nitrogen balance
Serum albumin
Vomiting
Electrolyte values
Intake and output measures
Temperature
Height, weight
Skin moist, dry; presence of lesions
Head, neck, hair
Nails, mouth, lips
Teeth, dentures, gums
Edema

■ PATTERN 3: ELIMINATION

Describes patterns of excretory function of the bowel, bladder, and skin.

Bladder

Subjective Data
Problem urinating
Frequency and urgency of urination
Daily fluid intake
Urinary tract infections

Objective Data
Presence of catheter, condom, ostomy
Palpable bladder
Palpable kidneys
Skin excoriation in genital area
Daily record of intake and output
Excessive perspiration

Bowel

Subjective Data
Use of laxatives
Constipation
Diarrhea
Use of stool softeners

Objective Data
Abdomen soft, tender, distended
Presence or absence of bowel sounds
Fistulas, ostomy
Drainage tubes
Skin excoriation
Roughage in diet

Skin

Subjective Data
Unpleasant odors
Pruritus
Presence of lesions

Objective Data
Unpleasant body odor
Drainage tubes
Draining skin lesions

■ PATTERN 4: ACTIVITY AND EXERCISE

Describes pattern of exercise and activity, respiratory and circulatory function.

Subjective Data
Breathing
Smoking
History asthma, bronchitis, or emphysema
Family history lung disease
Occupational hazards

Objective Data
Normal or abnormal lung sounds
Anteroposterior diameter (AP)
Chest tubes
Cough
Use of accessory muscles

Circulation

Subjective Data
Previous myocardial infarction, cerebrovascular accident
Pacemaker
Intermittent claudication
Use of medications affecting the peripheral vascular system

Objective Data
Normal or abnormal heart sounds
Capillary refill
Skin color
Lower extremity temperature and hair loss
Blood loss and use of replacement blood products
Central venous pressure (CVP)
Clotting factors
Serum glutamic pyruvic transaminase (SGOT)
Lactic dehydrogenase (LDH)

Mobility

Subjective Data
Verbalizes inability to climb stairs
Uses cane, walker
"I cannot do my activities of daily living anymore."
"I feel unsteady when walking."
"I do not have any energy."

Objective Data
Hand grip, reflexes
Ability to perform activities of daily living (ADL): feeding, bathing, toileting, bed mobility, dressing, shopping

Absence of body part
Prosthesis
Steady or unsteady gait, balance

■ PATTERN 5: SLEEP AND REST

Describes patterns of sleep, rest, and perception of energy level.

Subjective Data
Rested for daily activities
Drowsiness
Fatigue
Bedtime routine
Dreams or nightmares that interfere with sleep

Objective Data
Hypnotics, sedatives
Dark circles under eyes; ptosis (drooping eyelids)
Short attention span
Frequent yawning

■ PATTERN 6: COGNITIVE AND PERCEPTUAL

Describes patterns of hearing, vision, taste, touch, smell, pain perception, language, memory, and decision making.

Subjective Data
English as a second language
Educational level
Pain perception and management
Memory changes
Hearing aid or eyeglasses
Recent loss of body part or function
Rates pain on a scale of 0 to 10
Easiest method to learn (visual, hearing, doing)

Objective Data
Primary and secondary language spoken
Ability to follow directions
Decision-making ability
Level of consciousness
Neurologic examination
Oriented to time, place, person, and situation
Demonstrates knowledge of body parts

■ PATTERN 7: SELF-PERCEPTION AND SELF-CONCEPT

Describes attitudes about self and perception of abilities, self-worth, body image, feelings about self.

Subjective Data
Expressed desire to change self
Relaxed or nervous, rated on a scale of 1 to 5
Perceived powerlessness

Objective Data
Passive or assertive rated on a scale of 1 to 5
Nonverbal cues to altered self-esteem

■ PATTERN 8: ROLE AND RELATIONSHIP

Describes effectiveness of roles and relationships with family and others.

Subjective Data
Employment history
Effectiveness of relationships with family and others
Effect of role change on relationships
Financial concerns
Residence; homeless
Verbalizes physical or sexual abuse

Objective Data
Observed interaction with staff, family
Passive or aggressive behavior toward others
Participation of family in client's care
Diagram of family structure
Evidence of physical or sexual abuse

■ PATTERN 9: SEXUALITY AND REPRODUCTIVE

Describes actual or perceived satisfaction or problems with sexuality.

Subjective Data
Breast self-examination
Pruritus
Birth control measures
History of sexually transmitted diseases
History of sexual abuse

Objective Data
Breast examination
Genital lesions, pruritus, vaginal drainage, pain
Birth control measures
History of sexually transmitted disease
Laboratory results of Venereal Disease Research Laboratory (VDRL)
Human immunodeficiency virus (HIV) infection
Loss body part: breast, testicles, limb, eye
Evidence of sexual abuse

■ **PATTERN 10:** COPING AND STRESS TOLERANCE

Describes ability to manage stress and use of support systems.

Subjective Data
Use alcohol, illicit, and prescribed drugs to alleviate stress
Effect of illness on stress level
Rates anxiety on a scale of 0 to 5
Changes in family structure (death of parent, spouse, child)
Effect of community violence

Objective Data
Kinetic movements
Pacing

Adapted from: Gordon 1994.

No eye contact
Crying
Tone of voice
Facial expression

■ **Pattern 11:** VALUE AND BELIEF

Describes spirituality, values, belief system, and goals that guide the client's choices or decisions.

Subjective Data
Religious, cultural beliefs and practices
Attitude toward do not resuscitate (DNR) order
Perceived effect of disease on life's goals

Objective Data
Evidence of beliefs and values
Evidence of an advance directive or durable power of attorney

---

⬚ CASE STUDY #1: MR. JAMES HILL

Functional Health Patterns Approach to James Hill, a client with a medical problem (rheumatoid arthritis).

■ DEMOGRAPHIC DATA

Date of interview: 9/3/97
Client: James Hill
Address: 525 Westlady, Detroit, MI 48202
Telephone: 971-6288
Contact: Wife, Mildred
Address of contact: Same as client
Age Client: 64   Sex: Male   Race: Black
Educational background: High school
Religion: Baptist   Marital status: Married
Usual occupation: Photographer
Source of income: Self-employed
Insurance: Blue Cross/Blue Shield
Source of history: Client
Dominant language: English
Reliability of historian 4
(1 = unreliable; 4 = reliable)

■ ASSESSMENT USING GORDON'S 11 FUNCTIONAL HEALTH PATTERNS

• Health Perception-Health Management Pattern

History

Client's Responses "This is the worst attack of arthritis that I have had in the past 30 years. For the past 2 weeks, I have felt pain and noticed swelling, redness, and warmth over my knuckles. I have felt chills for the past 2 weeks. All of these problems started 3 months ago. I had an infected bunion on my left foot. The doctor lanced the bunion and pus poured out. The doctor put me on antibiotics."

Nurse's Observations Health record indicated that the client experienced an exacerbation of his rheumatoid arthritis signs and symptoms 8/18/97 and received a cortisone injection into his left wrist without relief of symptoms. On 8/18/97, the bunion was drained with copious amount purulent drainage. On

9/1/97, fluid cultured from client's painful left wrist. The health record revealed that on 8/12/97 methotrexate 2.5 mg orally was ordered for 5 days. On 8/18/97, the client was diagnosed with methotrexate toxicity, and the methotrexate was discontinued.

General Survey

Sitting on bed staring at floor during interview. Facial muscles taut. Holding sides of the bed for support. Warmth, redness, swelling right first and second metacarpal phalangeal joints and left bunion. Grimacing and moaning on movement of joints. Lesions throughout oral cavity. Temperature 101°F (R). Diaphoretic. Ulcer left foot crusty yellowish rim.

Past Health History

30-year history of rheumatoid arthritis; usually experiences three exacerbations every year. May take days to weeks to obtain pain relief with aspirin (ecotrin). Treated with antimalarials and gold in the past.

General Health

Rheumatoid arthritis major health problem. Denies shortness of breath (SOB). Decreased appetite and weight loss past month.

Prophylactic Physical and Dental

Annual examination by physician. Annual dental visits.

Surgical Procedures

Tonsillectomy 1940; implants secondary to removal of cataracts 1986.

Childhood Illnesses

Measles, whooping cough.

Immunizations

Received all childhood immunizations. Completed last tetanus 1985. Influenza immunization 1995.

Current Medications

Prescription
- Voltaren 50 mg Tabs 1 (po) tid
- Tylenol #3 Tabs 3–4/d (po) prn
- 9/3/97 Nafcillin g 2 IVP q4h started in emergency room. Heplock (heparin lock) in right forearm.

Nonprescription
- Ecotrin 325 mg Tabs 20–24 (po) qd for past 20 years.

Allergies

Methotrexate; grass.

Habits

46-year history of smoking one pack of cigarettes per day.

Family Health History

Maternal grandmother died at the age of 56 from complications of her diabetes mellitus. Father died cancer of gallbladder at age 76. Mother died of Alzheimer's disease at age 74. Cause of death of other grandparents unknown.

Social History

Photography business in client's home. Married 40 years. Wife 60 years old; works as a secretary. Five living children ages 37, 35, 30, 29, 27 years. Denies use of recreational drugs. Church functions constitute social activities.

Laboratory Findings 9/1/97

Culture
Fluid from left foot bunion positive for *Staphylococcus aureus*. White blood cells (WBCs) 11,000/µL (mm^3).

- **Nutritional-Metabolic Pattern**

History

Client's Responses "I prepare my breakfast and lunch, and my wife fixes dinner. I do not have food allergies. Now, I only eat a little food as nothing smells or tastes good, and my mouth is sore. When I saw the doctor 8/18/97, I could not smell or taste, and my mouth was full of sores. I was allergic to methotrexate. I cannot chew with all these sores so I puree all my food now. I rinse my mouth with water after each meal. I have lost weight this past month. I eat balanced meals. My wife makes sure there is food in the house. I have given up using salt. We cook with vegetable oil and use margarine. I feel chilly. I sweat a lot. I drink 2 juice glasses of water a day. I do not snack between meals."

Typical daily intake before mouth lesions

Breakfast
1 juice glass of orange juice, 1 cup of coffee, bowl of oatmeal with ¼ c. skim milk. One egg twice a week.
Lunch
Tuna-fish or ham sandwich on wheat toast, bowl of vegetable soup, fruit, 1 cup of coffee.

Dinner

Fish, rice, green vegetable, tossed salad with oil and vinegar dressing, 1 scoop of sherbet, 1 cup of decaffeinated coffee.

     Nurse's Observations At present, Mr. Hill eats pureed food. Social worker's note in the health record indicated that client had a food processor at home and pureed own food. Physician ordered low sodium (2 g), pureed diet. Ate 50% pureed lunch that consisted of peas, meat, fruit, and skim milk. Twenty-four hour fluid intake 980 mL.

Physical Examination

Height: 5'11" Large frame. Actual weight: 154 lb. Usual weight: 165 lb. Lost 10 lb. in past 6 months. Temperature 101°F (R). Skin hot to touch. Skin turgor: shape returned in 15 seconds. Diaphoretic. Positive subcutaneous nodules, firm on extremity surface. Hair sparse. No clubbing fingers. Ulcers throughout buccal mucosa; tongue and gums erythematous (red). Upper dentures; partial lower removed due to presence of lesions. Lips, tonsils, pharynx, speech within normal limits (WNL). Increased oral secretions. Halitosis.

Laboratory Findings 9/3/97

Blood

Serum albumin 3.5 g/dL
Serum potassium (K^+) 4.7 mEq/L
Serum sodium (Na^+) 133 mEq/L
Red blood cells (RBCs) 2.4 million/μL (mm3)
Hemoglobin (Hbg) 7.8 g/dL
Hematocrit (Hct) 22.3%
Glucose 105 mg/dL
Carbon dioxide (CO_2) 21.4 mEq/L
Chloride (Cl^-) 105 mEq/L
Calcium (Ca++) 9.4 mg/dL
Uric acid 1.32 mg/dL
Cholesterol 158 mg/dL

Urine

Specific gravity 1.026

• Elimination Pattern

History

Bowel

Client's Responses "I had a stool specimen taken a few weeks ago. The doctor said there was blood in it. I had blood in my stool several years ago. I move my bowels every morning after breakfast and I never take laxatives."

Physical Examination

Abdomen soft, nontender, nondistended, positive bowel sounds all 4 quadrants. Ability to control anal sphincter. No rectal lesions.

History

Urine

Client's Responses "I pass my water 8 to 10 times during the day. I have to go to the bathroom two to three times during the night. My stream of urine is slower."

Nurse's Observations The medical record indicated that the internist observed the stream and noted on the health record a decrease in the force of the urine stream. Client urinated twice during the 20-minute admission assessment.

Physical Examination

Kidney and bladder nonpalpable. No palpable masses.

Stool

Positive for occult blood

Laboratory Findings 9/3/97

Urinalysis

Pale yellow, clear. Specific gravity 1.026. Negative for leukocytes, nitrates, protein, glucose, ketones. Negative white blood cells (WBCs), red blood cells (RBCs), and casts.

Blood

Creatinine 1.1 mg/dL
Blood urea nitrogen (BUN) 44 mg/dL

• Activity and Exercise Pattern

History

Client's Responses "My arthritis is out of control. I am unable to do anything for myself. Please untie my shoes. My hands are swollen, and it is hard to move my fingers. I hold onto a chair when I walk around the house. The joints in my legs hurt when I stand or walk. I get tired when I make my breakfast and lunch. My wife opens all the food containers for me before she leaves for work. My feet have been puffy. My blood pressure runs high."

Physical Examination

Blood pressure (BP) 140/70, pulse 80 regular rhythm, respirations 20 regular rate. Extremities positive for subcutaneous nodules. Decreased range of motion (ROM) all joints. Abducts 15 degrees both shoulders.

Elbow flexion 70 degrees. Right wrist flexion 60 degrees. First and second metacarpophalangeal joints edematous, erythematous, tender and warm to touch. Weak hand grasp. Left hand in splint. Unable to undress self. Demonstrated unsteady balance and gait when walking. Walked 10 feet to bathroom and sat down twice en route. Both ankles 2+ edema and erythematous. Positive bunion left foot. No heart palpitations. Lungs clear to auscultation.

```
■ FUNCTIONAL LEVELS
Feeding      2    General mobility    3
Dressing     2    Bed mobility        2
Bathing      2    Home maintenance    3
Grooming     1    Cooking             3
Toileting    2    Shopping            3
```

```
■ FUNCTIONAL LEVEL CODES
Level 0:  Full self-care
Level 1:  Requires use of equipment or device
Level 2:  Requires assistance or supervision from
          another person
Level 3:  Requires assistance or supervision from
          another person and equipment or
          device
Level 4:  Is dependent and does not participate
```

```
■ SCALE FOR DESCRIBING EDEMA
1+   Barely detectable
2+   Indentation of less than 5mm
3+   Indentation of 5 to 10 mm
4+   Indentation of more than 10 mm
```

Laboratory Findings 9/3/97

Blood
Erythrocyte sedimentation rate (ESR) 59 mm/h
Rheumatoid factor 1:250 (latex fixation)

X-ray findings

Narrowing of joint space and bony erosions visualized.

● **Sleep and Rest Pattern**

History

Client's Responses "At home, I cannot sleep. I hurt all over. I get up in the morning and have difficulty moving. My wife helps me to a standing position. I have no energy. I do not believe in sleeping pills. I take two Ecotrin pills before I go to bed. I take an hour nap about 5 PM each day after all my business calls have stopped. My eyes feel tired. I am just too tired to talk."

Physical Examination

Stooped posture. Ptosis. Dark circles under eyes. Yawning throughout interview. Mispronounces words.

● **Cognitive and Perceptual Pattern**

History

Client's Responses "I am unable to taste or smell anything because of a reaction to my medication, methotrexate. I stopped taking methotrexate 2 weeks ago. I still cannot taste or smell, and the sores in my mouth hurt.

"My arthritis flares up several times a year and is usually relieved with Ecotrin. I hurt in all my joints. This time, the pain was not relieved with Ecotrin. During the past 2 weeks the pain has been worse than in the past 30 years. I usually have a dull, constant ache in all my joints. It feels like a knife is stabbing each joint. It hurts when you move my joints." Client taught to rate pain on a scale of 0 to 10. "I rate my pain an 8. I take Ecotrin 325 mg, 20 to 24 tablets a day to relieve my pain, and Tylenol #3 if I still hurt. I took 2 tablets of Tylenol #3 at 11 PM last night. Sometimes I get heartburn from taking too much Ecotrin."

Physical Examination

Hearing WNL. No ringing in ears. Wears reading glasses. Conjunctiva pink, moist. Cornea negative scleral icterus. Pupils equal, round, react to light and accommodation (PERRLA.) Nasal mucosa moist. Unable to identify smell on alcohol sponge when eyes closed. Unable to identify the taste of coffee. Lesions present oral cavity. Oriented to time, place, person, and situation (oriented ×4). Grimacing and moaning when each joint tested for ROM.

Laboratory Findings 9/3/97

Blood
Salicylate level 23 mg/dL

● **Self-perception and Self-concept Pattern**

History

Client's Responses "I am unable to run my photography business. Today, I work 4 hours a day answering the telephone. I was a track star in college and prided myself on my physical fitness. Now look at me. My body is bent over and my joints are large. I am not the man I used to be. I feel badly about my wife working because she is getting old. I cannot concentrate today. Please repeat your questions."

Nurse's Observations Spoke in halting, low voice. Nurse repeated interview questions, as client easily distracted. Looked at floor or wall during the interview. Stooped posture with little movement of body. Behavior rated a <u>2</u> on a scale of (1) passive to (5) assertive.

• Role and Relationship Pattern

History

Client's Responses "My wife earns the money now and pays all our bills. She works full time as a secretary. I used to earn all the money. She also cares for me. Our children call and visit at least every week. I have three sons and two daughters. They all help with my photography business and with the maintenance of the house. They have their own homes and families. I don't know how much longer they can help me."

Wife's Responses "I love to work. I was home caring for our children for 20 years. My husband needs to accept the fact that he cannot work anymore."

Nurse's Observations Wife accompanied client on admission. Wife holding client's hand during interview. Social worker's note on chart stated, "Observed husband and wife in problem-solving situation at home. Wife alert to the needs of husband. Children willingly assist with the business and chores."

• Sexuality and Reproductive Pattern

History

Client's Responses "We have 5 children and no problems with our sex life when we were young. I lost my interest in sex about 5 years ago. I am too tired and my joints hurt. I never asked my wife if this bothered her."

Nurse's Observations Client staring at floor. No eye contact with interviewer. Mumbling responses.

Physical Examination

Penis, urethra, scrotum, testes, epididymis, inguinal canal WNL. No masses. Prostate not enlarged. No penile drainage.

• Coping and Stress Pattern

History

Client's Responses "It took me 10 years before I accepted the fact that I had rheumatoid arthritis. I pace myself during the day. I answer the phone and book appointments for portraits and weddings. I realized a few years ago that I could no longer take wedding pictures so my oldest son does the weddings on the weekends. My children help out with the business. My oldest son is considering giving up his job at an automobile company and taking over the business for me. I can always act as a consultant. I do not smoke or drink anymore. I perform isometric exercises if I feel tense. Right now, I am worried about this infection and my joint pain. I rate my anxiety level <u>2</u> on a scale of 0 to 5."

Nurse's Observations No wringing hands or diaphoresis. Sitting quietly on bed. Facial muscles taut. Demonstrated isometric exercises. Social worker's note from home visit stated, "Children visit daily. Supportive family structure."

■ **ANXIETY RATING SCALE**
0 = No anxiety
1 = Verbalizes apprehension
2 = Increased level of concern
3 = Unfocused apprehension
4 = Sympathoadrenal response
5 = Panic

• Value and Belief Pattern

History

Client's Responses "My wife and I have belonged to the same Baptist church for our entire marriage. We go to church each Sunday, no matter how much my joints may be hurting. My faith in God has helped me through some painful days. We attend the potluck dinners on Friday nights and enjoy the fellowship. Our children and their families attend the church. It is wonderful seeing our 10 grandchildren. I assist with the food pantry on Saturdays and give food to folks in need. I enjoy helping other people."

Nurse's Observations Bible on bedside stand. Get-well cards taped to wall. Chaplain's pamphlet lying on bed. Smiled when talking about helping others.

EXERCISE 8–A: *IDENTIFICATION OF SUBJECTIVE DATA*

The purpose of Exercise 8–A is to aid in identifying the subjective data presented by the client, James Hill. Fill in the blanks below with subjective data from case study #1. Examples of subjective data from the case study are cited for each functional health pattern.

Pattern: Health Perception-Health Management, p. 84

1. "My knuckles are swollen."
2. _____
3. _____
4. _____
5. _____
6. _____
7. _____
8. _____

Pattern: Nutritional-Metabolic, p. 85

1. "I sweat a lot."
2. _____
3. _____
4. _____
5. _____
6. _____

Pattern: Elimination, p. 86

1. "I had blood in my stool several years ago."
2. _____
3. _____

Pattern: Activity-Exercise, p. 86

1. "I cannot do anything for myself."
2. _____
3. _____
4. _____
5. _____
6. _____
7. _____

Pattern: Sleep-Rest, p. 87

1. "My eyes feel tired."
2. _____
3. _____
4. _____

Pattern: Cognitive-Perceptual, p. 87

1. "I hurt in all my joints."
2. _____
3. _____
4. _____
5. _____

Pattern: Self-Perception and Self-Concept, p. 87

    1. "I am not the man I used to be." _____

    2. _____

    3. _____

    4. _____

    5. _____

Pattern: Role-Relationship, p. 88

    1. "My wife earns the money now . . .she also cares for me." _____

    2. _____

    3. _____

Pattern: Sexuality-Reproductive, p. 88

    1. "I lost my interest in sex about 5 years ago." _____

    2. _____

Pattern: Coping-Stress Tolerance, p. 88

    1. "I pace myself during the day." _____

    2. _____

    3. _____

    4. _____

Pattern: Value-Belief, p. 88

    1. "My faith in God has helped me." _____

    2. _____

    3. _____

    4. _____

EXERCISE 8–B: *IDENTIFICATION OF OBJECTIVE DATA*

The purpose of Exercise 8–B is to assist in identifying objective data demonstrated by the client, James Hill. Fill in the blanks with objective data noted in case study #1. Examples of objective data from the case study are cited for each functional health pattern.

Pattern: Health Perception-Health Management, p. 84

    1. Edema right first and second metacarpal phalanges. _____

    2. _____

    3. _____

    4. _____

    5. _____

    6. _____

    7. _____

    8. _____

Pattern: Nutritional-Metabolic, p. 85

    1. Skin turgor: shape returned in 15 seconds. _____

    2. _____

    3. _____

    4. _____

5. _____
6. _____

Pattern: Elimination, p. 86

1. <u>9/3/97 Melena in stool specimen.</u>_____
2. _____
3. _____

Pattern: Activity-Exercise, p. 86

1. <u>70 degree elbow flexion.</u>_____
2. _____
3. _____
4. _____
5. _____
6. _____
7. _____

Pattern: Sleep-Rest, p. 87

1. <u>Ptosis.</u>_____
2. _____
3. _____
4. _____

Pattern: Cognitive-Perceptual, p. 87

1. <u>Grimacing.</u>_____
2. _____
3. _____
4. _____
5. _____

Pattern: Self-Perception and Self-Concept, p. 87

1. <u>Spoke in halting, low voice.</u>_____
2. _____
3. _____
4. _____
5. _____

Pattern: Role-Relationship, p. 88

1. <u>Wife holding client's hand during interview.</u>_____
2. _____
3. _____

Pattern: Sexuality-Reproductive, p. 88

1. <u>Mumbling responses to questions.</u>_____
2. _____

Pattern: Coping-Stress Tolerance, p. 88

1. <u>Paces energy level.</u>_____
2. _____
3. _____
4. _____

Pattern: Value-Belief, p. 88

1. Bible on bedside stand. _____
2. _____
3. _____
4. _____

EXERCISE 8–C: *DATA VALIDATION*

The purpose of Exercise 8–C is to illustrate how to compare gathered data with accepted normal standards and values in order to determine the client's abnormal values. Listed below are subjective data (SD) validated by objective data (OD) from Mr. Hill's case study. Compare the client's subjective and objective values with accepted normal standards and values. A list of accepted normal values necessary to complete Exercise D is located in Appendix F.

Pattern: Health Perception/Management

1. Client value

SD: "My knuckles are swollen." _____

OD: Edema right first and second metacarpal phalanges. _____

Normal value: No edema metacarpal joints. _____

2. Client value

SD: " . . .pain . . .swelling, redness, warmth over knuckles." _____

OD: Warmth, redness, edema right metacarpal joints. _____

Normal value: _____

3. Client value

SD: "I had an infected bunion on my left foot." _____

OD: Ulcer left foot crusty yellowish rim. T 101°F(R). _____

Normal value: _____

4. Client value

SD: "I could not taste." _____

OD: Lesions throughout oral cavity. _____

Normal value: _____

5. Client value

SD: "I have felt chills." _____

OD: Temperature 101°F (R). Diaphoretic. Skin warm to touch. _____

Normal value: _____

6. Client value

SD: " . . .worst attack of arthritis in past 30 years." _____

OD: No relief symptoms with cortisone injection 8/18/97. _____

Normal value: _____

7. Client value

SD: "I am allergic to methotrexate."

OD: 8/12/97 Methotrexate 2.5 mg/d × 5days. D/C 8/18/97.

Normal value: _____

8. Client value

SD: "I have felt pain . . ."

OD: Facial grimacing; moaning upon joint movement.

Normal value: _____

Pattern: Nutritional-Metabolic

1. Client value

SD: "I sweat a lot."

OD: Skin turgor: Shape returned in 15 seconds.

Normal value: Prompt return of skin to normal shape.

2. Client value

SD: "I feel chilly."

OD: Temp. 101°F (R). Skin hot to touch. Diaphoretic.

Normal value: _____

3. Client value

SD: "I have lost weight."

OD: Weight loss 10 lb. past 6 months.

Normal value: _____

4. Client value

SD: "I drink two juice glasses of water a day."

OD: 24-hour oral fluid intake 980 mL.

Normal value: _____

5. Client value

SD: "I have given up using salt."

OD: Low-sodium, 2-G pureed diet ordered by physician.

Normal value: _____

6. Client value

SD: "My mouth is full of sores."

OD: Lesions throughout buccal mucosa.

Normal value: _____

Pattern: Elimination

1. Client value

SD: <u>"I had blood in my stool several years ago."</u>

OD: <u>9/3/97 lab. results revealed melena in stool specimen.</u>

Normal value: <u>No melena in stool.</u>

2. Client value

SD: <u>"I move my bowels every morning after breakfast and I never take laxatives."</u>

OD: <u>Abdomen nondistended, nontender.</u>

Normal value: _____

3. Client value

SD: <u>"My stream of urine is slower."</u>

OD: <u>Internist noticed decrease in force of urine stream.</u>

Normal value: _____

Pattern: Activity-Exercise

1. Client value

SD: <u>"I am unable to do anything for myself."</u>

OD: <u>70 degrees elbow flexion.</u>

Normal value: <u>150 degrees elbow flexion.</u>

2. Client value

SD: <u>"My hands are swollen . . .hard to move my fingers"</u>

OD: <u>Weak hand grasp. Swelling metacarpal phalangeal joints.</u>

Normal value: _____

3. Client value

SD: <u>"My feet have been puffy."</u>

OD: <u>Both ankles 2+ edema.</u>

Normal value: _____

4. Client value

SD: <u>"My blood pressure runs high."</u>

OD: <u>BP 140/70.</u>

Normal value: _____

5. Client value

SD: <u>"I get tired when I make my breakfast and lunch."</u>

OD: <u>Sat down twice en route bathroom 10 ft. from bed.</u>

Normal value: _____

6. Client value

SD: "My wife opens all the food containers . . ."

OD: Weak hand grasp.

Normal value: _____

7. Client value

SD: "I hold onto a chair when I walk around."

OD: Unsteady gait and balance when walking.

Normal value: _____

Pattern: Sleep-Rest

1. Client value

SD: "My eyes feel tired."

OD: Ptosis.

Normal value: _____

2. Client value

SD: "I cannot sleep."

OD: Dark circles under eyes. Ptosis.

Normal value: _____

3. Client value

SD: "I have no energy."

OD: Yawning throughout interview.

Normal value: _____

4. Client value

SD: "I am just too tired to talk."

OD: Mispronounces words.

Normal value: _____

Pattern: Cognitive-Perceptual

1. Client value

SD: "I hurt in all my joints."

OD: Grimacing.

Normal value: _____

2. Client value

SD: "This time, the pain was not relieved with Ecotrin."

OD: Order for Ecotrin 325 mg, 20–24 tablets/qd.

Normal value: _____

3. Client value

SD: "I rate my pain an eight." _____

OD: Client used scale of 0 to 10 to rate pain. Grimacing and moaning when joints tested for ROM. _____

Normal value: _____

4. Client value

SD: "It feels like a knife stabbing each joint." _____

OD: Grimacing and moaning on movement of joint. _____

Normal value: _____

5. Client value

SD: "I cannot taste or smell." _____

OD: Inability to identify smell alcohol and taste coffee. _____

Normal value: _____

Pattern: Self-Perception and Self-Concept

1. Client value

SD: "I am not the man I used to be." _____

OD: Spoke in halting, low voice. _____

Normal value: _____

2. Client value

SD: "My body is bent over and my joints are large." _____

OD: Stooped posture with little body movement. _____

Normal value: _____

3. Client value

SD: "I am unable to run my photography business." _____

OD: Behavior rated 2. _____

Normal value: _____

4. Client value

SD: "Please repeat your question." _____

OD: Easily distracted. Interview questions repeated. _____

Normal value: _____

5. Client value

SD: "I feel badly about my wife working . . ." _____

OD: Looked at floor or wall during interview. _____

Normal value: _____

Pattern: Role-Relationship

1. Client value

SD: "My wife earns the money now . . .she also cares for me."

OD: Wife holding client's hand.

Normal value:

2. Client value

SD: "[Children] help with my photography business and . . .house."

OD: Social workers noted children assisted with business.

Normal value:

3. Client value

SD: "My husband needs to accept the fact . . .cannot work . . ."

OD: Wife and client observed in problem-solving situation.

Normal value:

Pattern: Sexuality-Reproductive

1. Client value

SD: "I never asked my wife if it bothered her."

OD: Mumbling responses to questions.

Normal value:

2. Client value:

SD: "I am too tired and my joints hurt."

OD: No eye contact with interviewer.

Normal value:

Pattern: Coping-Stress Tolerance

1. Client value

SD: "I pace myself during the day."

OD: Paces energy level.

Normal value:

2. Client value

SD: "I am worried about this infection and joint pain."

OD: Facial muscles taut.

Normal value:

3. Client value

SD: " . . .10 years accept . . .rheumatoid arthritis."

OD: No wringing hands. Rated anxiety level 2 on a scale of 0 to 5.

Normal value:

4. Client value

SD: <u>"I perform isometric exercises if I feel tense."</u>

OD: <u>Demonstrated isometric exercises.</u>

Normal value: _____

Pattern: Value-Belief

1. Client value

SD: <u>"My faith in God has helped me."</u>

OD: <u>Bible on bedside stand.</u>

Normal value: _____

2. Client value

SD: <u>"I enjoy helping other people."</u>

OD: <u>Many get-well cards posted on the wall.</u>

Normal value: _____

3. Client value

SD: <u>"We go to church each Sunday . . ."</u>

OD: <u>Chaplain's pamphlet lying on bed.</u>

Normal value: _____

4. Client value

SD: <u>"I assist with the food pantry and give food to folks in need."</u>

OD: <u>Smiled when talking about helping others.</u>

Normal value: _____

EXERCISE 8–D: *IDENTIFICATION OF DYSFUNCTIONAL HEALTH PATTERNS*

The purpose of Exercise 8–D is to identity dysfunctional health patterns in the case study subject, James Hill. Subjective and objective data were compared with normal values in Exercise 8–C. Based on your findings in Exercise 8–C, identify the dysfunctional patterns, that is, the patterns demonstrating the majority of abnormal values and standards. Mark (X) for YES or NO. YES indicates the pattern is dysfunctional; NO, the pattern is not dysfunctional. Write your rationale, the critical thinking involved, to support your judgment. Rationale is the logical or fundamental reason for selecting a response. Citing related literature may be required to support the stated critical thinking (rationale). An example is provided for the Health Perception and Health Management pattern.

Pattern: Health Perception-Health Management
Dysfunctional   YES <u>X</u>   NO ___
Critical thinking: <u>Subjective data (increase in joint pain) and objective data (elevated WBC) manifested the signs and symptoms of inflammation and infection, resulting in an exacerbation of the rheumatoid arthritis joint pain.</u>

Pattern: Nutritional-Metabolic
Dysfunctional   YES ____   NO ____
Critical thinking:

_____
_____
_____
_____

Pattern: Elimination
Dysfunctional   YES ____   NO ____
Critical thinking:

_____
_____
_____
_____

Pattern: Activity-Exercise
Dysfunctional   YES ____   NO ____
Critical thinking:

_____
_____
_____
_____

Pattern: Sleep-Rest
Dysfunctional   YES ____   NO ____
Critical thinking:

_____
_____
_____
_____

Pattern: Cognitive-Perceptual
Dysfunctional   YES ____   NO ____
Critical thinking:

_____
_____
_____
_____

Pattern: Self-Perception and Self-Concept
Dysfunctional   YES ____   NO ____
Critical thinking:

_____
_____
_____
_____

Pattern: Role-Relationship
Dysfunctional   YES ___   NO ___
Critical thinking:

_____
_____
_____
_____

Pattern: Sexuality-Reproductive
Dysfunctional   YES ___   NO ___
Critical thinking:

_____
_____
_____
_____

Pattern: Coping-Stress Tolerance
Dysfunctional   YES ___   NO ___
Critical thinking:

_____
_____
_____
_____

Pattern: Value-Belief
Dysfunctional   YES ___   NO ___
Critical thinking:

_____
_____
_____
_____

EXERCISE 8–E: *FORMULATING A THREE-PART NURSING DIAGNOSIS*

The purpose of Exercise 8–E is to illustrate how to formulate a three-part nursing diagnosis. The health patterns listed below were identified as dysfunctional in Exercise 8–D. For each dysfunctional pattern, formulate a minimum of one nursing diagnostic statement for the client, James Hill. Refer to the nursing diagnoses listed under each functional health pattern in Appendix C. Refer to Appendix B for definitions of nursing diagnoses to determine the appropriate nursing diagnosis. An example of a nursing diagnosis for the dysfunctional health pattern Health Perception-Health Management is cited below.

Health Perception-Health Management

1. **Nursing diagnostic statement for dysfunctional pattern: Health Perception-Health Management**
   Nursing diagnostic label: <u>Altered protection</u> _____
   Related to: <u>immunosuppression</u> _____
   Defining characteristics (as evidenced by): <u>warmth, redness, edema left wrist/foot; 9/1/97 WBC 11,000;</u>
   <u>bunion culture positive *Staphylococcus aureus.*</u> _____
2. **Nursing diagnostic statement for dysfunctional pattern: Nutritional-Metabolic**
   Nursing diagnostic label: _____
   Related to: _____

Defining characteristics (as evidenced by): _____

_____

_____

_____

3. **Nursing diagnostic statement for dysfunctional pattern: Activity-Exercise**

Nursing diagnostic label: _____

_____

Related to: _____

_____

Defining characteristics (as evidenced by): _____

_____

_____

_____

4. **Nursing diagnostic statement for dysfunctional pattern: Sleep-Rest**

Nursing diagnostic label: _____

_____

Related to: _____

_____

Defining characteristics (as evidenced by): _____

_____

_____

_____

5. **Nursing diagnostic statement for dysfunctional pattern: Cognitive-Perceptual**

Nursing diagnostic label: _____
Related to: _____

_____

Defining characteristics (as evidenced by): _____

_____

_____

_____

6. **Nursing diagnostic statement for dysfunctional pattern: Self-Perception and Self-Concept**

Nursing diagnostic label: _____
Related to: _____
Defining characteristics (as evidenced by): _____

_____

_____

_____

7. **Nursing diagnostic statement for dysfunctional pattern: Sexuality-Reproductive**

Nursing diagnostic label: _____

_____

Related to: _____

_____

Defining characteristics (as evidenced by): _____

_____

_____

_____

EXERCISE 8–F: *RANKING NURSING DIAGNOSES*

The purpose of Exercise 8–F is to illustrate the ranking of nursing diagnoses in order of their importance, starting with #1 as the highest priority (life-threatening) to the lowest priority (self-actualization). Gordon (1994, p. 205) states to "check to see if some problems do not require immediate treatment. Are they low priority?" This thought process reflects Maslow's Hierarchy of Needs. For this exercise, nursing diagnosis will be ranked based on Maslow's hierarchy. Rank the nursing diagnoses identified in Exercise 8–E for the James Hill case study, in order of high, medium, to low priority. An example is provided based on Exercise 8–E.

NURSING DIAGNOSIS	MASLOW'S NEEDS	RANKING
1. Altered protection	Physiologic	High
2.		
3.		
4.		
5.		
6.		
7.		

EXERCISE 8–G: *FORMULATING OUTCOME CRITERIA*

The purpose of Exercise 8–G is to illustrate formulation of outcomes for the James Hill case study. Write outcome criteria for the four nursing diagnoses with the highest priority identified in Exercise 8–F. An example is cited below.

1. Nursing diagnosis: Altered protection

   Outcome criteria

   Subject: Client

   Measurable verb: will demonstrate

   Outcome: changing of dressing on left bunion

   Criteria: accurately

   Target time: by 9/20/97

2. Nursing diagnosis:

   Outcome criteria

   Subject:

   Measurable verb:

   Outcome:

   Criteria:

   Target Time:

3. Nursing diagnosis:

   Outcome criteria

   Subject:

   Measurable verb:

   Outcome:

   Criteria:

   Target time:

4. Nursing diagnosis: _____

   Outcome criteria

   Subject: _____

   Measurable verb: _____

   Outcome: _____

   Criteria: _____

   Target time: _____

EXERCISE 8–H: *WRITING NURSING INTERVENTIONS*

The purpose of Exercise 8–H is to illustrate the writing of nursing interventions for outcomes. Using the outcomes listed in Exercise 8–G, write one nursing intervention for each outcome criterion.

1. Outcome criterion: <u>Client and wife will demonstrate changing of dressing on left bunion accurately by 9/20/97.</u>

   Nursing intervention

   Date written: <u>9/8/97</u>

   Measurable verb: <u>teach</u>

   Subject: <u>client and wife</u>

   Outcome: <u>dressing change on bunion</u>

   Target time: <u>by 9/5/97</u>

   Signature: <u>Jolene Vezzetti, RN</u>

2. Outcome criterion: _____

   _____

   Nursing intervention

   Date written: _____

   Measurable verb: _____

   Subject: _____

   Outcome: _____

   Target time: _____

   Signature: _____

3. Outcome criterion: _____

   _____

   Nursing intervention

   Date written: _____

   Measurable verb: _____

   Subject: _____

   Outcome: _____

   Target time: _____

   Signature: _____

4. Outcome criterion: _____
_____

Nursing intervention

Date written: _____

Measurable verb: _____

Subject: _____

Outcome: _____

Target time: _____

Signature: _____

EXERCISE 8–I: WRITING A NURSING CARE PLAN CASE STUDY #1: MR. JAMES HILL

The purpose of Exercise 8–I is to illustrate the writing of a nursing care plan for Case Study #1. Using the following format, select one high-priority nursing diagnosis from Exercise 8–F p. 102. Based on the nursing diagnosis that you chose, include the appropriate subjective data, objective data, dysfunctional health pattern, outcome criteria, nursing diagnostic statement, cause and defining characteristics, interventions, and the critical thinking to support each nursing order. Additional outcome criteria and nursing orders may be written.

ASSESSMENT	NURSING DIAGNOSTIC STATEMENT	OUTCOMES
Subjective Data Exercise 8–A, p. 89	*Nursing Label* _____	1: Subject: _____
_____	_____	Measurable Verb: _____
_____	*Related to*	Outcome: _____
_____	_____	Criterion: _____
Objective Data Exercise 8–B, p. 90	_____	Target Time: _____
_____	_____	2: Subject: _____
_____	*Defining Characteristics (as evidenced by)*	Measurable Verb: _____
_____	_____	Outcome: _____
DYSFUNCTIONAL HEALTH PATTERN:	_____	Criterion: _____
_____	_____	Target Time: _____
_____	_____	

OUTCOMES (CONT)

3: Subject: _____

Measurable Verb: _____

Outcome: _____

Criterion: _____

Target Time: _____

NURSING INTERVENTIONS FOR

Outcome 1:
Date:
Measurable Verb: _____
Subject: _____
Outcome: _____
Target Time: _____
Signature: _____

Outcome 2:
Date:
Measurable Verb: _____
Subject: _____
Outcome: _____
Target Time: _____
Signature: _____

Outcome 3:
Date:
Measurable Verb: _____
Subject: _____
Outcome: _____
Target Time: _____
Signature: _____

CRITICAL THINKING FOR

Nursing Intervention
_____
_____
_____
_____
_____

Nursing Intervention
_____
_____
_____
_____
_____

Nursing Intervention
_____
_____
_____
_____
_____

EXERCISE 8–J: _IDENTIFICATION OF INDEPENDENT NURSING ACTIONS_

The purpose of Exercise 8–J is to illustrate how to write independent nursing actions. Review the nursing interventions listed in Exercise 8–H. List below the nursing interventions that represent independent nursing actions.

1. <u>Teach the client to change dressing on bunion.</u> _____
2. _____
3. _____
4. _____

EXERCISE 8–K: _WRITING NURSES' NOTES_

The purpose of Exercise 8–K is to illustrate how to write accurate nurses' notes. In this exercise, write a narrative nurse's note, a SOAP note, and a Focus note for the James Hill case study, based on the following situation. Refer to the example for narrative notes on p. 66, SOAP notes p. 66, and Focus notes p. 68.

Situation for Exercise 8–K

On 9/8/97, at 1230, Janet Jones, RN, arrives in Mr. Hill's room and the following conversation occurs.

Mr. Hill:	"I am having pain in all my joints. They really hurt."
Nurse:	"How long have you been in pain? Would you please rate your pain on a scale of 0 to 10, with 0 being no pain and 10 excruciating pain."
Mr. Hill:	"I rate my pain an 8."
Nurse:	"What do you take to relieve the pain at home?"
Mr. Hill:	"I take 20 to 24 tablets of Ecotrin a day at home. I need some Tylenol #3 for this pain."

Nurse:	(Observes that Mr. Hill is moaning, facial muscles taut. BP 160/80. Pulse 100). "Is the pain throbbing or sharp?"
Mr. Hill:	"It feels like a knife is stabbing each joint."

Date 9/8/97   Time 1245

Nurse:	(Administers Tylenol #3, 2 tablets, orally to Mr. Hill. Nurse returns at 1315 to check the effectiveness of the medication).

Time 1315

Nurse:	"How would you rate your pain now, Mr. Hill?" (Nurse notes no grimacing or moaning. BP 140/80. P 80).
Mr. Hill:	"I feel better. I rate my pain a 4."
Nurse:	"I am going to teach you distraction techniques to help alleviate your pain."

EXERCISE 8–K-1: WRITING *NARRATIVE* NURSES' NOTES

Date _____ Time _____ Nurse's Note _____

_____
_____
_____
_____
_____
_____
_____
_____
_____
_____
_____
_____
_____
_____
_____
_____
_____
_____
_____
_____
_____

EXERCISE 8–K-2: WRITING *SOAP* NURSES' NOTES

Date _____ Time _____ Nurse's Note _____

S: _____
_____
_____

O: _____
_____
_____

A: _____
_____

P: _____
_____
_____

EXERCISE 8–K-3: WRITING *FOCUS* NURSES' NOTES

	Date	Time	Focus Nurse's Note

DATA:

_____

_____

_____

_____

_____

ACTION:

_____

_____

_____

RESPONSE:

_____

_____

_____

TEACHING:

_____

_____

_____

_____

EXERCISE 8–L: *EVALUATION OF OUTCOMES*

The purpose of Exercise 8–L is to evaluate the achievement of outcomes noted on the nursing care plan. In Exercise 8–G, outcomes were identified for James Hill. Based on the information related in the paragraph below, write an evaluation of whether the outcomes listed in Exercise 8–G were resolved.

Scene 9/28/97:

Mr. Hill is scheduled for discharge 9/30/97. He demonstrated the ability to walk 50 feet using a walker. The edema, redness, and tenderness in joints have subsided. His joints remain positive for subcutaneous nodules. Limited ROM of all joints continues. Demonstrated the ability to assist with bathing, dressing, and feeding self. Ate 100% of his meals. Stated, "I can taste the food now." No lesions present in his mouth. Skin turgor returns immediately. Ulcer left foot dry and culture negative. Wife demonstrated ability to change dressing on bunion using aseptic technique. Hemoglobin 14 g/dL. Hematocrit 40%. Visiting nurse to see client 10/1/97.

1. Outcome criterion: <u>Client will demonstrate changing of dressing on bunion accurately by 9/20/97.</u>
   Resolved: YES ___X___   NO _____
   Evaluation: <u>Wife demonstrated changing of sterile dressing on bunion accurately. Client unable to perform</u>
   <u>task because of limited joint mobility.</u>
2. Outcome criterion: _____
   _____
   Resolved: YES _____   NO _____
   Evaluation: _____
   _____
3. Outcome criterion: _____
   _____
   Resolved: YES _____   NO _____
   Evaluation: _____
   _____
   _____
   _____
4. Outcome criterion: _____
   _____
   Resolved: YES _____   NO _____
   Evaluation: _____
   _____
   _____

✔ CORRECT RESPONSES TO EXERCISES BASED ON FUNCTIONAL HEATH PATTERNS AND CASE STUDY #1, JAMES HILL

EXERCISE 8–A: *IDENTIFICATION OF SUBJECTIVE DATA*

Pattern: Health Perception-Health Management

1. <u>"My knuckles are swollen."</u>
2. <u>" . . .pain . . .swelling, redness, warmth over</u>
   <u>knuckles."</u>
3. <u>"I had an infected bunion on my left foot."</u>
4. <u>"I could not taste."</u>
5. <u>"I have felt chills for the past 2 weeks."</u>
6. <u>" . . .worst attack of arthritis . . .in past 30</u>
   <u>years."</u>
7. <u>"I was allergic to methotrexate."</u>
8. <u>"I have felt pain . . . ."</u>

Pattern: Nutritional-Metabolic

1. <u>"I sweat a lot."</u>
2. <u>"I feel chilly."</u>
3. <u>"I have lost weight."</u>
4. <u>"I drink 2 juice glasses of water a day."</u>
5. <u>"I have given up using salt."</u>
6. <u>"My mouth is sore."</u>

Pattern: Elimination

1. <u>"I had blood in my stool several years ago."</u>
2. <u>"I move my bowels every morning."</u>
3. <u>"My stream of urine is slower."</u>

Pattern: Activity-Exercise

1. <u>"I am unable to do anything for myself."</u>
2. <u>"My hands are swollen . . .hard to move my</u>
   <u>fingers."</u>
3. <u>"My feet have been puffy."</u>
4. <u>"My blood pressure runs high."</u>
5. <u>"I get tired when I make my breakfast and</u>
   <u>lunch."</u>
6. <u>"My wife opens all the food containers . . ."</u>
7. <u>"I hold onto a chair when I walk around . . ."</u>

Pattern: Sleep-Rest

1. <u>"My eyes feel tired."</u>
2. <u>"I cannot sleep."</u>
3. <u>"I have no energy."</u>
4. <u>"I am just too tired to talk."</u>

Pattern: Cognitive-Perceptual

1. "I hurt in all my joints."
2. "This time, the pain was not relieved with Ecotrin."
3. "I rate my pain an 8."
4. "It feels like a knife is stabbing each joint."
5. "I still cannot taste or smell."

Pattern: Self-Perception/Self-Concept

1. "I am not the man I used to be."
2. "My body is bent over and my joints are large."
3. "I am unable to run my photography business."
4. "Please repeat your questions."
5. "I feel badly about my wife working . . ."

Pattern: Role-Relationship

1. "My wife earns the money now . . .she . . . cares for me."
2. "[Children] help with my photography business and . . .house."
3. "My husband needs to accept the fact he cannot work . . ."

Pattern: Sexuality-Reproductive

1. "I lost my interest in sex about 5 years ago."
2. "I am too tired and my joints hurt."

Pattern: Coping-Stress Tolerance

1. "I pace myself during the day."
2. "I am worried about this infection and joint pain."
3. ". . .10 years [to accept] . . .rheumatoid arthritis."
4. "I perform isometric exercises if I feel tense."

Pattern: Value-Belief

1. "My faith in God has helped me . . ."
2. "I enjoy helping other people."
3. "We go to church each Sunday . . ."
4. "I assist with the food pantry [and help] folks in need."

EXERCISE 8–B: *IDENTIFICATION OF OBJECTIVE DATA*

Pattern: Health Perception-Health Management

1. Edema right first and second metacarpal phalanges.
2. Warmth, redness, edema right metacarpal joints.

3. Ulcer left foot crusty yellowish rim.
4. Lesions throughout oral cavity.
5. Temperature 101°F (R). Diaphoretic. Skin warm to touch.
6. No relief symptoms with cortisone injection 8/18/97.
7. Methotrexate 2.5 mg/d × 5 days. Discontinued 8/18/97.
8. Grimacing; moaning on joint movement.

Pattern: Nutritional-Metabolic

1. Skin turgor: shape returned in 15 seconds.
2. Temperature 101°F (R). Skin hot to touch. Diaphoretic.
3. Weight loss 10 lb. past 6 months.
4. 24-hour oral fluid intake 980 mL.
5. Low-sodium 2 g pureed diet ordered by physician.
6. Lesions throughout buccal mucosa.

Pattern: Elimination

1. 9/3/97 Melena in stool specimen.
2. Abdomen nondistended, nontender.
3. Internist noted decrease in force urine stream.

Pattern: Activity-Exercise

1. 70 degree elbow flexion.
2. Weak hand grasp. Swelling metacarpal phalangeal joints.
3. Both ankles 2+ edema.
4. BP 140/90.
5. Sat down twice en route bathroom 10 ft. from bed.
6. Weak hand grasp.
7. Unsteady gait and balance when walking.

Pattern: Sleep-Rest

1. Ptosis.
2. Dark circles under eyes. Ptosis.
3. Yawning throughout interview.
4. Mispronounces words.

Pattern: Cognitive-Perceptual

1. Facial grimacing.
2. Ecotrin 325 mg, 20-24 tablets/qd.
3. Grimacing and moaning when joints tested for ROM.
4. Grimacing and moaning upon movement joint.
5. Inability to identify smell of alcohol or taste coffee.

Pattern: Self-Perception and Self-Concept

1. Spoke in halting, low voice.
2. Stooped posture with little body movement.
3. Behavior rated 2.
4. Easily distracted. Interview questions repeated.
5. Looked at floor or wall during interview.

Pattern: Role-Relationship

1. Wife holding client's hand during interview.
2. Social worker noted children assist with business.
3. Wife and client observed in problem-solving situation.

Pattern: Sexuality-Reproductive

1. Mumbling responses to questions.
2. No eye contact with interviewer.

Pattern: Coping-Stress Tolerance

1. Paces energy level.
2. Facial muscles taut.
3. No wringing hands. Rated anxiety level 2 on scale 0 to 5.
4. Demonstrated isometric exercises.

Pattern: Value-Belief

1. Bible on bedside stand.
2. Many get-well cards posted on the wall.
3. Chaplain's pamphlet lying on bedside stand.
4. Smiled when talking about helping others.

EXERCISE 8–C: *DATA VALIDATION*

Pattern: Health Perception-Management

1. Client value

SD: "My knuckles are swollen."

OD: Edema right first and second metacarpal phalanges.

Normal value: No edema of metacarpal joints.

2. Client value

SD: ". . .pain . . .swelling, redness, warmth over knuckles."

OD: Warmth, redness, edema right metacarpal joints.

Normal value: No signs or symptoms of inflammation.

3. Client value

SD: "I had an infected bunion on my left foot."

OD: Ulcer left foot crusty yellowish rim. T 101°F (R).

Normal value: No crusting, signs or symptoms of infection.

4. Client value

SD: "I could not taste."

OD: Lesions throughout oral cavity.

Normal value: Sense of taste; numerous taste buds tongue.

5. Client value

SD: "I felt chills."

OD: Temperature 101°F (R). Diaphoretic. Skin warm to touch.

Normal value: Temperature for age 98.6°F/ 99.6°F (R).

6. Client value

SD: " . . .worst attack of arthritis . . .in past 30 years."

OD: No relief symptoms with cortisone injection 8/18/97.

Normal value: Anti-inflammatory action of cortisone.

7. Client value

SD: "I am allergic to methotrexate."

OD: 8/12/91 Methotrexate 2.5 mg/d (po) → 5days D/C 8/18/97.

Normal value: No allergic reaction to methotrexate.

8. Client value

SD: "I have felt pain . . ."

OD: Grimacing; moaning on joint movement.

Normal value: Full ROM without joint pain.

Pattern: Nutritional-Metabolic

1. Client value

SD: "I sweat a lot."

OD: Skin turgor: Shape returned in 15 seconds.

Normal value: Prompt return of skin to normal position.

2. Client value

SD: "I feel chilly."

OD: Temp. 101°F (R). Skin hot to touch. Diaphoretic.

Normal value: No temperature, skin warm, no diaphoresis.

3. Client value

SD: "I have lost weight."

OD: Weight loss 10 lb. past 6 months.

Normal value: Maintain normal weight.

4. Client value

SD: "I drink 2 juice glasses of water a day."

OD: 24-hour oral fluid intake 930 mL

Normal value: 1200 mL oral/2500 mL total fluid intake/24h.

5. Client value

SD: "I have given up using salt."

OD: Low-sodium, 2g pureed diet ordered by physician.

Normal value: 1100-3300 mg sodium/d.

6. Client value

SD: "My mouth is full of sores."

OD: Lesions throughout buccal mucosa.

Normal value: No lesions buccal mucosa.

Pattern: Elimination

1. Client value:

SD: "I had blood in my stool several years ago."

OD: 9/3/97 Stool positive occult blood.

Normal value: No melena.

2. Client value

SD: "I move my bowels every morning."

OD: Abdomen nondistended, nontender.

Normal value: Nondistended, nontender abdomen

3. Client value

SD: "My stream of urine is slower."

OD: Internist noticed decrease in force urine stream.

Normal value: Detrusor muscles able to contract.

Pattern: Activity-Exercise

1. Client value

SD: "I cannot do anything for myself."

OD: 70 degrees elbow flexion.

Normal value: 150 degrees elbow flexion.

2. Client value

SD: "My hands are swollen . . .hard to move my fingers."

OD: Weak hand grasp; swelling metacarpal phalanx joints.

Normal value: No swelling joints; ability to grasp firmly; 3.

3. Client value

SD: "My feet have been puffy."

OD: Both ankles 2+ edema.

Normal value: No edema present.

4. Client value

SD: "My blood pressure runs high."

OD: BP 140/70.

Normal value: BP 120/80 for age.

5. Client value

SD: "I get tired when I make my breakfast and lunch."

OD: Sat down twice en route bathroom 10 ft. from bed.

Normal value: Ability to perform ADL.

6. Client value

SD: "My wife opens all the food containers . . ."

OD: Weak hand grasp.

Normal value: Firm hand grasp; ability to perform ADL.

7. Client value

SD: "I hold onto a chair when I walk around . . ."

OD: Unsteady gait and balance when walking.

Normal value: Steady gait and balance when walking.

Pattern: Sleep-Rest

1. Client value

SD: "My eyes feel tired."

OD: Ptosis.

Normal value: No drooping of eyelids.

2. Client value

SD: "I cannot sleep."

OD: Dark circles under eyes; ptosis.

Normal value: No dark circles under eyes; no ptosis.

3. Client value

SD: "I have no energy."

OD: Yawning throughout interview.

Normal value: Sufficient energy to perform ADL.

4. Client value

SD: "I am just too tired to talk."

OD: Mispronounces words.

Normal value: Ability to communicate clearly.

Pattern: Cognitive-Perceptual

1. Client value

SD: "I hurt in all my joints."

OD: Grimacing.

Normal value: No joint pain.

2. Client value

SD: "This time, the pain was not relieved with Ecotrin."

OD: Order for Ecotrin 325 mg, 20-24 tablets/qd.

Normal value: Ecotrin 2.6–5.2 g/d orally (po) divided doses.

3. Client value

SD: "I rate my pain an 8."

OD: Grimacing, moaning when joints tested for ROM.

Normal value: Full ROM without pain.

4. Client value

SD: "It feels like a knife is stabbing each joint."

OD: Grimacing, moaning on movement joint.

Normal value: Full ROM without pain.

5. Client value

SD: "I still cannot taste or smell."

OD: Inability to identify smell alcohol and taste coffee.

Normal value: Sense of taste and smell intact.

Pattern: Self-Perception and Self-Concept

1. Client value

SD: "I am not the man I used to be."

OD: Spoke in halting, low voice.

Normal value: Feelings of self-worth.

2. Client value

SD: "My body is bent over and my joints are large."

OD: Stooped posture with little body movement.

Normal value: Erect posture; no enlarged joints.

3. Client value

SD: "I am unable to run my photography business."

OD: Behavior rated 2.

Normal value: Behavior (1) passive to (5) assertive

4. Client value

SD: "Please repeat your questions."

OD: Easily distracted; interview questions repeated.

Normal value: Ability to concentrate on task at hand.

5. Client value

SD: "I feel badly about my wife working . . ."

OD: Looked at floor or wall during interview.

Normal value: Positive feelings of human value.

Pattern: Role-Relationship

1. Client value

SD: "My wife earns the money now . . .she also cares for me."

OD: Wife holding client's hand.

Normal value: Caring relationship.

2. Client value

SD: "[Children] help with my photography business and . . .house."

OD: Social worker noted children assist with business.

Normal value: Supportive family relationships.

3. Client value

SD: "My husband needs to accept the fact . . . cannot work . . . "

OD: Wife and client observed in problem-solving situation.

Normal value: Use cognitive skills to deal with stressor.

Pattern: Sexuality-Reproductive

1. Client value

SD: "I never asked my wife if it bothered her."

OD: Mumbling responses to question.

Normal value: Ability to express self to loved ones.

2. Client value

SD: "I am too tired and my joints hurt."

OD: No eye contact with interviewer.

Normal value: Ability to express self to interviewer.

Pattern: Coping-Stress Tolerance

1. Client value

SD: "I pace myself during the day."

OD: Paces energy level.

Normal value: Time management to conserve energy.

2. Client value

SD: "I am worried about this infection and joint pain."

OD: Facial muscles taut.

Normal value: Toned facial muscles; ability to express fears.

3. Client value

SD: ". . .10 [years to accept] . . . rheumatoid arthritis."

OD: No wringing hands; rated anxiety level 2 on a scale of 0 to 5.

Normal value: Recognition of limitations, impact disease.

4. Client value

SD: "I perform isometric exercises if I feel tense."

OD: Demonstrated isometric exercises.

Normal value: Isometric exercise increase muscle strength.

Pattern: Value-Belief

1. Client value

SD: "My faith in God has helped me."

OD: Bible on bedside stand.

Normal value: Belief system provides meaning to life.

2. Client value

SD: "I enjoy helping other people."

OD: Many get-well cards posted on the wall.

Normal value: Social support system for times of stress.

3. Client value

SD: "We go to church each Sunday . . ."

OD: Chaplain's pamphlet lying on bedside stand.

Normal value: Belief system provides support.

4. Client value

SD: "I assist with the food pantry and [help] folks in need."

OD: Smiled when talking about helping others.

Normal value: Helping others increases self-worth.

EXERCISE 8–D: *IDENTIFICATION OF DYSFUNCTIONAL HEALTH PATTERNS*

Pattern: Health Perception-Health Management
Dysfunctional   YES __X__   NO _____
Critical Thinking: Subjective data (increase in joint pain) and objective data (elevated WBC) demonstrated the signs and symptoms of inflammation and infection, resulting in exacerbation of the rheumatoid arthritis.

Pattern: Nutritional-Metabolic
Dysfunctional   YES __X__   NO _____
Critical Thinking: Demonstrated decreased skin turgor with 24-hour fluid intake of 980 mL less than normal 1200 mL/24 h. Lesions throughout buccal mucosa interfered with taste sensation and mastication of food.

Pattern: Elimination
Dysfunctional   YES __X__   NO _____
Critical Thinking: 9/3/97 stool specimen positive for melena. Decrease in force urine. Majority values within normal limits.

Pattern: Activity-Exercise
Dysfunctional   YES __X__   NO _____
Critical Thinking: Subjective data (lack of energy) and objective data (unsteady gait, limited ROM, and enlargement of joints) validate client's inability to perform ADL without assistance. Elevated blood pressure and 2+ edema both feet may indicate cardiovascular problem.

Pattern: Sleep-Rest
Dysfunctional   YES __X__   NO _____
Critical Thinking: Verbal expressions of fatigue and inability to sleep. Change from optimal adult sleep pattern of 7 to 8 hours for age resulting in lack of energy to perform ADL.

Pattern: Cognitive-Perceptual
Dysfunctional   YES __X__   NO _____
Critical Thinking: Verbalized increased pain in all joints. Pain elicited upon movement of joints. Perceived no relief with pain medication. Present pain management ineffective in alleviating pain. Diminished sense of taste and smell.

Pattern: Self-Perception and Self-Concept
Dysfunctional   YES __X__   NO _____
Critical Thinking: Low self-esteem resulting from decrease in physical abilities, changes in body function and appearance. Inability to manage own business. Decreased attention span; behavior passive.

Pattern: Role-Relationship
Dysfunctional   YES __X__   NO _____
Critical Thinking: Wife earns sufficient income to meet family's financial needs. Client demonstrated ability to verbalize feelings regarding the change in the roles of family members. Wife and children provide family support system. Majority of findings WNL.

Pattern: Sexuality-Reproductive
Dysfunctional   YES __X__   NO _____
Critical Thinking: Inability to verbalize perceived changes in sexuality pattern with partner. Progression of client's disease process has prevented the continuation of previous sexual expressions. No evidence of counseling in this area.

Pattern: Coping-Stress Tolerance
Dysfunctional   YES _____   NO __X__
Critical Thinking: Ability to identify fears and concerns. Recognizes limitations. Implemented strategies to reduce stress. Family support system in place. Majority of findings within normal limits.

Pattern: Value-Belief
Dysfunctional   YES _____   NO __X__
Critical Thinking: Practices beliefs and values that also serve as a coping strategy. Ability to extend self to others in need. Social support system in place. Wife, husband, and children share common beliefs and values. Majority findings within normal limits.

EXERCISE 8–E: *FORMULATING A THREE-PART NURSING DIAGNOSTIC STATEMENT*

1. Nursing diagnosis: Altered protection related to immunosuppression as evidenced by WBC 11,000; culture positive *Staphylococcus aureus;* heat, redness, and swelling joints.

2. Nursing diagnosis: Alteration in oral mucous membrane related to drug reaction as evidenced by presence of buccal lesions, decreased sense of taste, oral pain.

3. Nursing diagnosis: Impaired physical mobility: Level I related to uncompensated musculoskeletal impairment as evidenced by unsteady gait, limited range of motion, decreased muscle strength.

4. Nursing diagnosis: Sleep pattern disturbance related to physical discomfort as evidenced by dark circles under eyes, ptosis, verbalized feelings of fatigue.

5. Nursing diagnosis: Pain related to chronic physical disability as evidenced by facial grimacing and verbalization of pain on movement of joints; rated pain 8 on scale 0 to 10.

6. Nursing diagnosis: Self-esteem disturbance related to loss of significant role as evidenced by decrease in physical abilities, stooped posture, verbalized changes in body appearance.

7. Nursing diagnosis: Altered sexuality patterns related to change in body functions as evidenced by limitation and pain of physical movement, inability to discuss perceived changes with wife.

EXERCISE 8–F: *RANKING NURSING DIAGNOSES*

NURSING DIAGNOSIS	MASLOW'S NEEDS	RANKING
1. Altered protection	Safety	High
2. Pain	Physiologic	High
3. Altered oral mucous membrane	Physiologic	Medium
4. Impaired physical mobility	Physiologic	Medium
5. Sleep-pattern disturbance	Physiologic	Medium
6. Self-esteem disturbance	Self-esteem	Low
7. Altered sexuality patterns	Love, belonging	Low

EXERCISE 8–G: *FORMULATING OUTCOMES*

1. Outcome
   Subject: Client and wife
   Measurable verb: will demonstrate
   Outcome: changing of dressing on left bunion
   Criteria: accurately
   Target time: by 9/20/97
2. Outcome
   Subject: Client
   Measurable verb: will practice
   Outcome: slow, rhythmic breathing
   Criteria: independently before pain rating reaches 4.
   Target Time: by 9/4/97
3. Outcome
   Subject: Client
   Measurable verb: will rinse
   Outcome: buccal mucosa, tongue, gums with saline
   Criteria: after each meal and at bedtime
   Target time: by 9/5/97

4. Outcome
   Subject: Client
   Measurable verb: will walk
   Outcome: safely with a walker
   Criteria: 20 feet 4 times a day
   Target time: by 9/14/97

EXERCISE 8–H: *WRITING NURSING INTERVENTIONS*

1. Nursing Intervention
   Measurable verb: Teach
   Subject: client and wife
   Outcome: aseptic dressing change on bunion
   Target time: by 9/5/97
   Signature: Janet Jones, RN
2. Nursing Intervention
   Measurable verb: Teach
   Subject: client
   Outcome: pain reduction through rhythmic breathing
   Target time: 9/3/97
   Signature: Janet Jones, RN
3. Nursing Intervention
   Measurable verb: Demonstrate
   Subject: to client
   Outcome: medical aseptic techniques used to cleanse mouth
   Target time: 9/3/97
   Signature: Janet Jones, RN
4. Nursing intervention
   Measurable verb: Demonstrate
   Subject: to client and wife
   Outcome: safe ambulating techniques with a walker
   Target time: by 9/5/97
   Signature: Janet Jones, RN

EXERCISE 8-1: *WRITING A NURSING CARE PLAN*

Part 1: Using altered protection as the high-priority nursing diagnosis

ASSESSMENT

Subjective Data
"My knuckles are swollen."
"I have pain, redness, and warmth over my knuckles."
"I had an infected bunion on my left foot."

Objective Data
WBC 11,000
Culture positive staphylococcus
Edema, redness metacarpal phalanges

DYSFUNCTIONAL HEALTH PATTERN
Health Management-Health Perception

OUTCOME CRITERIA

1. Client will demonstrate changing of dressing on left bunion accurately by 9/29/97.

2. Client will verbalize signs and symptoms of infection unassisted by 9/20/97.

3. Client will verbalize the role of protein in tissue regeneration accurately by 9/10/97.

NURSING DIAGNOSTIC STATEMENT

Nursing Diagnostic Label
Altered protection

Related to
immunosuppression

Defining Characteristics (as evidenced by)
increase in WBC, edema, redness joints, positive culture staphylococcus

NURSING INTERVENTIONS
Outcome 1:
A: Teach client and wife to change dressing on bunion by 9/20/97. Cyndie Smith, RN

Outcome 2:
B: Teach client and wife early signs of inflammation and infection, by 9/1/97. Cyndie Smith, RN

Outcome 3:
C: Teach the client and wife the basic 4 food groups by 9/12/97. Cyndie Smith, RN

CRITICAL THINKING
Nursing Intervention A:
Medical asepsis limits the number of microorganisms and their spread.

Nursing Intervention B:
Open wounds are portals of entry for microorganisms. Hand washing is the most effective means of controlling the spread of microorganisms.

Nursing Intervention C:
A balanced diet supplies essential proteins and vitamins to build new tissue.

Part 2: Using pain as high-priority nursing diagnosis

NURSING DIAGNOSTIC STATEMENT

ASSESSMENT

Nursing Diagnostic Label
Pain

Subjective Data
"It feels like a knife is stabbing each joint."
"I rate my pain an 8."
"This time, the pain was not relieved with Ecotrin."
"It hurts when you move my joints."

Related to
chronic disease

Defining characteristics (as evidenced by)
verbalizations of pain on joint movement, rated pain intensity an 8, grimacing

Objective Data
Grimacing
Moaning when each joint tested for ROM
Salicylate level 23mg/dL

DYSFUNCTIONAL HEALTH PATTERN
Cognitive-Perceptual

OUTCOME CRITERIA

1. Client will verbalize pain rating before-pain reaches a 4 by 9/3/97.

2. Client will practice slow rhythmic breathing independently by 9/4/97.

3. Client will realistically identify factors that exacerbate the pain by 9/4/97.

NURSING INTERVENTIONS

Outcome 1:
A: Teach the client to rate pain intensity on scale of 0–10 by 9/3/97. Cyndie Smith, RN

Outcome 2:
B: Teach the client slow rhythmic breathing by 9/4/97. Cyndie Smith, RN

Outcome 3:
C: Evaluate client's pain management by 9/4/97. Cyndie Smith, RN

CRITICAL THINKING

Nursing Intervention A:
The intensity or severity of pain is subjective. The pain rating scale is designed to assist clients in describing the intensity of their pain.

Nursing Intervention B:
Relaxation techniques are effective in reducing anxiety, muscle tension, and dissociation from the pain.

Nursing Intervention C:
Establishing a pain management program will lead to realistic pain control goals.

EXERCISE 8–J: *INDEPENDENT NURSING ACTIONS*

1. Teach the client and wife to change dressing on bunion.
2. Teach client pain reduction through rhythmic breathing.
3. Demonstrate medical aseptic technique used to cleanse mouth.
4. Demonstrate safe ambulating techniques with a walker.

EXERCISE 8–K-1: *WRITING NARRATIVE NURSES' NOTES*

Date	Time	
9/4/97	1230	Nurse's note: Pain
		Stated, "I am having pain in all my joints. I rate my pain an 8 on scale 0 to 10. I take Ecotrin 20 to 24 tablets a day at home. I need some Tylenol #3 for this pain. It feels like a knife is stabbing each joint." Moaning, facial muscles taut. BP 160/80 P 100 R 22. Janet Jones, RN
9/4/97	1245	Tylenol #3 Tab. 2 given po. Janet Jones, RN
9/4/97	1315	Nurses note: Pain
		Stated, "I feel better. I rate my pain a 4 on scale 0 to 10." BP 140/80, P 80, R 18. No grimacing. Taught distraction techniques to alleviate pain. Janet Jones, RN

EXERCISE 8–K-2: *WRITING SOAP NURSES' NOTE*

Date	Time	Nurse's Note: Pain
9/4/97	1230	S: "I am having pain in my joints. I rate my pain an 8 on scale 0 to 10. I take Ecotrin 20 to 24 tablets day at home. I need some Tylenol #3 for this pain. It feels like a knife is stabbing each joint." O: Moaning. Facial muscles taut. BP 160/80 P 100, R 22. A: Pain persists P: Teach client to request pain medication before pain reaches rating of 4. Teach client non-pharmacologic interventions to reduce pain such as imagery, rhythmic breathing. Janet Jones, RN

9/4/97	1245	I: Administered Tylenol #3 2 Tabs (po). Taught rhythmic breathing to help relieve pain. Janet Jones, RN
9/4/97	1315	E: Rated pain 4. Practicing slow, rhythmic breathing. No grimacing or moaning. BP 40/80 P 80 R: Teach wife to observe husband's pain management. Janet Jones, RN

EXERCISE 8–K-3: *WRITING FOCUS NURSES' NOTES*

Date	Time	
9/4/97	1230	Focus Nurse's Note: Pain
		DATA: Stated, "I am having pain in all my joints. I rate my pain an 8 on scale 0 to 10. I take Ecotrin 20 to 24 tablets a day at home. I need some Tylenol #3 for this pain. It feels like a knife is stabbing each joint." Moaning. Facial muscles taut. BP 160/80. P 100. R 22. Janet Jones, RN
9/4/97	1245	ACTION: Tylenol #3 Tabs 2 (po) given. Janet Jones, RN
9/4/97	1215	RESPONSE: Stated, "I feel better, I rate my pain a 4." No grimacing or moaning. BP 140/80. P 80 R 18. TEACHING: Taught distraction techniques for alleviation of pain. Janet Jones, RN

EXERCISE 8–L: *EVALUATING THE ACHIEVEMENT OF OUTCOMES*

1. Outcome: Client and wife will demonstrate changing of dressing on bunion accurately by 9/20/97.
   Resolved: YES __X__ NO _____
   Evaluation: Wife demonstrated changing of sterile dressing on bunion accurately. Client unable to perform task as result limited joint mobility.
2. Outcome: Client will practice slow, rhythmic breathing independently before pain rating reaches 4 by 9/4/97.
   Resolved: YES __X__ NO _____
   Evaluation: Client observed practicing slow, rhythmic breathing independently an average of 4 times during the AM and PM shifts and used during the night as sleep aid. Client verbalized, "For the majority of the time, I keep

my pain rating to a 3 using the rhythmic breathing."

3. Outcome: Client will rinse buccal mucosa, tongue, and gums with saline after each meal and at bedtime by 9/5/97.
   Resolved: YES ___X___   NO _____
   Evaluation: Client observed rinsing mouth with saline after each meal and at bedtime. Because limited joint mobility, client expressed verbal difficulty in handling the glass. On observation, client was able to put glass to mouth, rinse mouth, and expectorate saline without assistance. Buccal lesions persist. Rinses will be continued.

4. Outcome: Client will walk with a walker unassisted 20 feet, 4 times a day by 9/14/97.
   Resolved: YES ___X___   NO _____
   Evaluation: By 9/14/97, client demonstrated the ability to walk with a walker unassisted, 20 feet, 4 to 6 times a day. Client verbalized a feeling of increased strength in quadriceps muscles.

Case Study Using a Body Systems Approach

The current emphasis on interdisciplinary collaboration among health care providers has increased the use of a body systems approach to assessment. The body systems model (medical model) has been used for years by physicians, nurse practitioners, and other health care providers as the framework for collecting data from clients. Preprinted assessment and reassessment forms may use a body system format. One such format for collecting data is presented below. As students progress through the nursing curriculum, they put into practice more aspects of the body system assessment.

A Body Systems Approach for Obtaining the History and Physical Information for an Adult Client

Dates

Record:

- date of history
- age
- sex
- race
- place of birth
- marital status
- occupation
- dominant language
- religion

Source of history

Note the source of the history and whether the information was obtained from:

- client
- family
- friends
- client's medical records
- a referral letter from a physician

Reliability of the source

Determine the reliability (credibility) of responses from the client, family, and friends. Rate the reliability of the source on a scale of 1 to 4 with 1 = unreliable source and 4 = reliable source.

Chief complaint(s)

Write within quotation marks the words the client used to describe his or her problems ("I am short of breath all the time").

Present illness

- Write in chronologic order the sequence of events leading to the problem.
- Organize the data to include the onset of the problem, the setting in which it developed, its manifestations, and any treatments to date.
- Describe the seven attributes of the symptoms in terms of:
  - location
  - quality
  - quantity or severity
  - timing (onset, duration, and frequency)
  - the setting in which symptoms occur
  - factors that have aggravated or relieved symptoms
  - associated manifestations

- Record the client's perception of the effects the chief complaint has had on his or her life (relationships with others; ability to work and perform desired activities).

Past history

- General state of health from the client's point of view ("I have been healthy until now")
- Childhood illnesses (measles, chickenpox)
- Adult illnesses (pneumonia, pyelonephritis)
- Psychiatric illnesses (depression, post-traumatic stress disorder, paranoia)
- Accidents and injuries (including fractures, falls at home)
- Surgery (appendectomy, cholecystectomy)
- Emergency room visits and hospitalizations not already described
- Current health status ("I have been sick on and off the past 2 weeks")
- Current health promotion practices (annual physical examinations, dental examination, effect of cultural practices on seeking care from health care providers)
- Current medications, including the influence of cultural practices on health care in the use of home and folk remedies (herbal teas), nonprescription drugs (aspirin), prescription drugs (digoxin)
- Environmental allergies (ragweed, medications, food)
- Tobacco (including number of cigarettes smoked per day)
- Alcohol (type, amount per day, last drink), drugs (what, such as marijuana, and last use), caffeine (coffee or tea, coca cola, cocoa, and number of cups per day)
- Diet (whether low cholesterol, low salt, low purine)
- Screening tests (vision, hearing, mammogram, tuberculin)
- Immunizations (tetanus, influenza)
- Sleep patterns (5 hours of uninterrupted sleep each night without the use of sedatives; use of comfort measures to induce sleep; or use of sedatives or hypnotics to induce sleep)
- Exercise (daily walks, roller blading, jogging) and leisure activities (bingo, reading)
- Environmental hazards (working in an environment where toxic fumes are prevalent or where there are flying chips of metal)
- Use of safety measures (work goggles, back supports, fitted breathing masks, steel-toe safety shoes)

Family history

- Age, health, or cause of death of each immediate family member (parents, siblings, spouse, children); for example, maternal grandfather died of a heart attack at age 67
- Occurrence within the family of diabetes, heart disease, high cholesterol, high blood pressure, stroke, kidney disease, tuberculosis, cancer, arthritis, anemia, allergies, asthma, headaches, epilepsy, mental illness, alcoholism, drug addiction, or symptoms similar to those of the client

Psychologic history

Describe the client as a person (agitated or relaxed; passive or aggressive; evaluate ability to deal with daily stressors).

Home situation and relationship with others

Describe family structure including who lives with the client and who assists when illness occurs. Evidence of physical or sexual abuse (ecchymotic areas over body; fractured bones; verbalization of abuse).

Daily life

Describe a typical day in the life of the client.

Significant life experiences

- Education
- Military service
- Job history
- Financial situation
- Marriage
- Recreation
- Retirement

Cultural, religious, and spiritual beliefs

Perceptions of health, illness, and treatment. Influence of nontraditional medicine (acupressure, acupuncture) on health and illness practices.

Review of systems

General review includes height and weight compared with average for frame, recent weight change (as in cancer, hyperthyroidism, anorexia nervosa), weakness (may indicate low potassium level), fatigue (may signal low hemoglobin), fever.

- **Skin** (note rashes, sores, lumps, dryness, color changes in hair or nails, presence of lice or scabies)
- **Head** (note headache, injury, lumps)

- **Eyes** (note vision, glasses or contact lenses, last eye examination, pain, redness, excessive tearing, double vision, blurred vision)
- **Ears** (note ability to hear, dizziness, ringing in the ears, earaches, discharge, use of hearing aids)
- **Nose and sinuses** (note frequent colds; nasal stuffiness, drainage, nosebleeds)
- **Mouth and throat** (note condition of teeth and gums, bleeding gums, dentures, last dental examination, sore throats, hoarseness)
- **Neck** (note swollen glands, goiter, pain or stiffness in the neck)
- **Breast** (note lumps, pain, nipple discharge, history of self-examination)
- **Respiratory** (note cough, spitting up blood, crackling sounds (rales), wheezing (rhonchi), color of sputum, last chest x-ray film)
- **Cardiac** (history of heart problems or high blood pressure, chest pain, rapid heart rate, shortness of breath)
- **Gastrointestinal** (note problem swallowing, heartburn, appetite, anorexia, nausea, vomiting, frequency of bowel movements, change in bowel habits, rectal bleeding, tarry stools, constipation, diarrhea, evidence of bulimia)
- **Urinary** (note frequency, polyuria, nocturia, burning, hematuria, urgency, dribbling, infections)
- **Genital** Males (note hernias, discharge, sexually transmitted disease).
  Females (note age at menarche, periods, dysmenorrhea, menopause, discharge, sores, sexually transmitted diseases, number of pregnancies)
- **Peripheral vascular** (note leg cramps, varicose veins, intermittent claudication, extremity numbness and tingling)
- **Musculoskeletal** (note muscle or joint pains, arthritis, backache, limitation of movement and ADL, gait, balance, evidence of injury)
- **Neurologic** (note vertigo, headaches, fainting, blackouts, seizures, weakness, paralysis, numbness or loss of sensation, tingling, involuntary movements)
- **Hematologic** (note anemia, easy bruising, past transfusions and any reactions).
- **Endocrine** (note hyperthyroidism, hypothyroidism, heat or cold intolerance, diabetes, excessive thirst or hunger)
- **Psychiatric** (note nervousness, tension, paranoia, bulimia, mood, depression, memory)

S CASE STUDY #2: MRS. JUDITH SMITH

Body Systems Approach to a Client with a Surgical Problem (carcinoma left breast, stage I with subsequent mastectomy).

■ DEMOGRAPHIC DATA

Date of History 9/3/97, 1100

Client: Judith Smith

Address: 1621 Hampton, Seminole, Florida 34642

Contact: Husband, Charles Smith

Address of contact: Same as client

Age: 49   Sex: Female   Race: White

Religion: Catholic   Marital status: Married

Usual occupation: Medical records technician for a hospital

Source of income: Salary from employment. Husband is an accountant

Medical Insurance: Health Alliance Plan (HAP)

Source of History

Client

Dominant Language

English

Reliability of Historian 4

"My name is Judith Smith. It is Wednesday, September 3, 1997. I am at the Urban Hospital and scheduled to have my breast removed tomorrow, September 4, 1997." Oriented to time, place, person, and situation (oriented ×4).

Clear about her symptoms and when they began.

Chief Complaint

"I have a lump in my left breast."

Present Illness

"I noticed the lump in my left breast during my monthly breast self-examination 6 months ago. I kept putting off going to the doctor. Finally, I went to the doctor 2 months ago. A biopsy was performed at that time. The doctor told me the tumor was malignant. I go to surgery tomorrow to have my left breast removed and maybe some nodes. I had been very healthy until this happened to me. I expect to be cured of cancer after this surgery. I am concerned my husband will find me unattractive after the mastectomy. We use to have sex at least once a week. Now we rarely have sex. My husband says he is too tired and does not want to talk about sex. Sex is not the most important thing. I know he loves me as he is thoughtful."

Frown on face when discussing sexual relations.

Past History

General state of health
"Other than my migraine headaches, I have been in good health until the lump in my breast developed. My usual blood pressure is 120/80. I started menstruating at 13 years and my periods last 3 days. My last period was August 25, 1997. I do not have any vaginal discharge. I had 2 pregnancies and 2 children. I use oral contraceptives."

Childhood illness
None stated

Adult Illnesses
"I have had migraine headaches for the past 20 years. I get a migraine once a month. My head has been pounding for the past 2 weeks. I am having a migraine headache right now. It is a steady throbbing pain around my left eye. I rate the intensity a 7 on a scale of 0 to 10. I take 1 ergotamine tablet when my headache begins and it usually works. I forgot to bring my ergotamine with me and I need some medication. I get a migraine when I have been under a lot of stress. I get nauseated with the headaches and feel nauseated right now. I turned the lights off and pulled the shades because the light hurts my eyes."

Lying quietly in bed with eyes closed when interviewer arrived in room. Rubbing forehead over left eye. Radio and television off.

Psychiatric illness
None stated

Accidents or injuries
"I fell on the tennis court in 1985 and broke my left wrist and arm. I have full use of the arm now and have no problem playing tennis."

Surgery
"I had a breast biopsy performed July 1997 in the Urban Hospital's Outpatient Surgery Clinic."

Hospitalizations
None stated

Current health status
"I have no pain or tenderness in my left breast. I found the lump while performing my monthly breast exam. This is upsetting to me. My heart feels like it is racing, which is a new feeling, as I have had no cardiac problems, no chest pain, no heart flutters or racing of my heart in the past. I never had rheumatic fever, phlebitis, numbness, tingling or pain in my legs. I have had no spitting up of blood, and there has been no change in frequency or amount of urine."

"I have had a problem with constipation for the past 2 months. I decided to take Metamucil every night. The doctor prescribed Colace once a day. My last bowel movement was last night, and the stool was hard. I have stopped eating salads at lunch and dinner. I am too nauseated. My internist does a rectal exam at my annual physical. I usually urinate six times a day. I never have bladder infections. I do not have pain or discomfort when I urinate. I never get up at night to urinate."

Current Health Promotion Practices
"Since 1986, I have had a physical examination once a year, and my last exam was 2 months ago. I have had a mammogram and a Pap smear annually for the past 11 years. I see the dentist every 6 months. I shower and wash my hair every day, and I scrub my teeth after every meal. I exercise daily and usually eat balanced meals. I play tennis and take long walks to relieve my tension."

Current medications
Prescription
- Colace 100 mg/d PO qd
- ergotamine 2 mg PO at onset migraine
- temazepam 30 mg Tab. 1 PO hs prn
- diphenhydramine (Benadryl) 25 mg PO q6h prn
- metaproterenol (Alupent) 0.65mg 2 inhalations q4h prn

Nonprescription
- Calcium 500 mg/d
- Multivitamins Tab 1/d

Allergies
"I have hay fever and if it gets bad, I develop asthma. I wheeze when I have an asthma attack and

get short of breath. My mother and maternal grandmother had asthma. My eyes and nose have been itching and watering this week. I take Benadryl for my hay fever and took Benadryl 25 mg before I came to the hospital today. I also took 2 whiffs of Alupent in my nebulizer this morning because I started to sound wheezy. The Alupent stopped the wheezing for a few hours. I do not want my asthma to begin, especially since I will be going to surgery. I do not have any food allergies."

Tobacco use

"I never smoked."

Alcohol, drugs, caffeine

"I drink five cups of coffee per day and more when I get nervous. I do not drink alcohol or use recreational drugs."

Diet

"I have lost 10 pounds in 3 weeks. I usually eat three balanced meals a day and drink two juice glasses of water a day. I pack a lunch for work. I buy all the groceries and cook all the meals. My husband does not help. I feel nauseated and too upset to eat today. I ate a bowl of soup for dinner at 6 o'clock last night. In the past month, I have had heartburn at least once a day. I do not use diuretics. I feel chilly."

Ate 25 percent of food on lunch tray. Full pitcher of water on bedside stand.

■ **TYPICAL DAILY INTAKE**

Breakfast: 1 glass orange juice, 1 cup coffee, and 1 slice wheat toast with jam.

Lunch: Ham on white bread, cookies, and 2 cups of coffee.

Dinner: Steak, baked potato, rolls, butter, chocolate cake, and 2 cups coffee.

Evening snack: Candy.

Screening tests

"I have no problems with hearing, and I wear glasses to read."

Immunizations

"Usual childhood immunizations such as tetanus, measles, whooping cough, diphtheria, polio, and smallpox."

Sleep patterns

"I usually sleep 8 hours each night. Sometimes I take a 15-minute rest when I arrive home from work. Since I received the biopsy results 2 months ago, I only sleep 2 to 3 hours. I usually get up and read the newspaper. The doctor ordered sleeping medication for me. I am tired at work lately. My eyelids feel heavy."

Dark circles under eyes. Rubbing eyes during interview. Ptosis.

Exercise

"I play tennis once a week, and I usually walk two miles each evening."

Environmental hazards

None stated

Safety measures

"I wear glasses at work to read fine print."

Family History

"My father is alive, 75 years old, and has coronary artery disease. I am not worried, even though my maternal grandmother died of breast cancer at age 49 and my mother died of breast cancer at age 53.

Psychological History

"I am not concerned about money, but I am concerned about my radical mastectomy scheduled for tomorrow. I hope I can wear a bikini after this surgery. My husband thinks I have a great figure. I told him about my surgery but he will not talk about it. We travel a lot and I think he is afraid our trips will be cancelled by my surgery. He will be here shortly. I rate my anxiety level a 2 on a scale of 0 to 5. I hope this surgery will not change my relationship with my husband. I am so nervous. I wish my husband would hurry up and get here."

Grimacing. Wringing hands. Decreased attention span. Nurse allowed client a 30-minute rest period due to pain; nurse returned to complete the interview.

Home Situation and Relationships with Others

"My husband is 52 years old. He works full-time as an accountant. We have two children ages 21 and 23. Our children are both in college and visit on holidays. We talk with them each weekend on the telephone. I love my husband and children. My husband and I live in a ranch home in a small town. Our social life consists of attending office parties at our places of employment and church functions. My father lives 25 miles from my house and joins us for

Sunday dinners. At home, I go for walks just to get rid of all my anger.

"I anticipate no problems after my surgery. This will be a quick surgery and recovery period. I plan to be home 2 days after my mastectomy and return to work 2 weeks from the day of surgery. My church group said they would bring dinners over for the first week after my discharge."

Daily Life

"I work full-time as a medical records technician at a hospital."

Significant Life Experiences

Background

"I have an associate degree in medical records. Learning new things has been easy for me."

Job History

"I have worked full-time for 10 years."

Military service

None stated.

Financial situation

"I am not concerned about money but I am concerned about my radical mastectomy scheduled for tomorrow."

Married

"I have been married 27 years."

Recreation

"I play tennis once a week, and I walk 2 miles each evening."

Retirement

"I plan to retire when I reach 62 years old, and my husband will retire when he is 65."

Religious and Spiritual Beliefs

"I am a Catholic and have gone to church every Sunday for years. I asked my priest why did I have to get cancer? He did not respond. I believe that God is punishing me for something. It is not fair. I have lived a good life. I told my husband that I would not go to church anymore."

Review of Systems

General

Actual height 5′6″. Actual weight 110 lb. Small frame. T 99.2°F (PO), P 90. Yawning through-

out interview. Medical record reveals previous annual physical examinations from 1986–1997. Blood pressure readings of 120/80, pulse 78, respirations 16.

Skin   No body odor. Skin, hair, and nails clean. Skin pale, moist. Skin intact integrity. Skin warm to the touch. Skin turgor: shape returned in 10 seconds. Hair evenly distributed. Scalp hair silky, thick texture. Hair combed neatly. Nail beds pink. Positive blanching sign. Nails manicured.

Eyes   Pupils equal round react to lightand accommodation (PERRLA). Redness and lacrimation (tearing) eyes. Visual acuity tests reveal able to read newsprint with glasses.

Ears   Hearing acuity tests reveal normal voice tones audible; hears whispered, spoken words.

Nose/sinuses   Nasal turbinates pale, edematous; watery nasal drainage.

Mouth/throat   Teeth: 32 adult teeth. No partial plates. Oral cavity: lips, breath, tongue, tonsils, pharynx, speech and salivary gland within normal limits (WNL). No difficulty swallowing.

Neck   Palpable neck and shoulder muscles.

Breast   One-inch scar on left breast. Left breast lump palpable, nontender, dimpling of skin over upper-outer sector. Hard, irregular, poorly delineated, nonmobile lump. No nipple discharge. No palpable lumps in right breast.

Respiratory   Respirations 24, regular rate and rhythm. No shortness of breath (SOB). No dyspnea upon exertion. No nasal flaring or use of accessory muscles. Auscultation of chest revealed minimal wheezing on expiration both lungs.

Cardiac   Blood pressure (BP) 150/80 sitting; 146/80 lying. Apical rate 90, regular rhythm at rest. No pedal edema. No jugular vein distention.

Gastrointestinal   Abdomen nontender, moderately distended, positive bowel sounds all quadrants. Rectal deferred. No palpable masses.

Urinary Genital   Kidney and bladder nonpalpable. No vaginal drainage or lesions. Genitalia examination deferred.

Peripheral Vascular   Blanching sign: immediate capillary refill nail beds. Extremities warm to the touch. Palpable pedal pulses.

Peripheral Pulses
- Temporal-4 bilateral
- Carotid-4 bilateral
- Brachial-4 bilateral
- Radial-4 bilateral
- Femoral-4 bilateral
- Popliteal-4 bilateral
- Posterior tibial-4 bilateral
- Dorsalis pedis-4 bilateral

Periperal Pulse Scale
0-Absent
1-Markedly diminished
2-Moderately diminished
3-Slightly diminished
4-Normal

Musculoskeletal Slight hand tremor. Firm muscle tone. Strength equal all extremities. Range of motion (ROM) within normal limits. Wrist 80–90 degree flexion and extension. Gait steady. Posture well balanced.

Functional Levels

Feeding	0	General mobility	0
Dressing	0	Bed mobility	0
Bathing	0	Home maintenance	0
Grooming	0	Cooking	0
Toileting	0	Shopping	0

Functional Level Codes
Level 0:   Full self-care
Level 1:   Requires use of equipment or device
Level 2:   Requires assistance or supervision from another person
Level 3:   Requires assistance or supervision from another person, equipment or device
Level 4:   Is dependent and does not participate

Neurologic Alert. No facial drooping. Handgrasps equal. Speech clear. Learns quickly. Ability to verbalize recent and past events. Denies problems with swallowing.

Pain Rating Intensity Scale 0–10

0 = no pain	6 = moderate pain
1 = slight pain	7 = disabling pain
2 = slight pain	8 = disabling pain
3 = mild pain	9 = disabling pain
4 = mild pain	10 = Unbearable pain
5 = moderate pain	

Mrs. Smith rated the pain from her migraine headache a 7, on a scale of 0–10.

Endocrine No dysfunction noted

Psychiatric/Psychologic Changed position from bed to chair 5 times during interview. Speaking in a loud, abrupt voice. Constantly talking. Eyes darting around the room. Facial muscles taut. Face flushed. Began crying during interview. Wringing hands. Began pacing floor. Husband not present. Smiled when talking about husband and children.

Anxiety Rating Scale
0 = No anxiety
1 = Verbalizes apprehension
2 = Increased level of concern
3 = Unfocused apprehension
4 = Sympathoadrenal response
5 = Panic

Mrs. Smith rated her anxiety level a 2 on a scale of 0–5.

Laboratory Findings 9/3/97

Blood chemistry	Serum albumin 5.2 g/dL
	Serum glucose 105 mg/dL
	Blood urea nitrogen (BUN) 8 mg/dL
	Sodium (Na$^+$) 150 mEq/L
	Chloride (Cl$^-$) 90 mEq/L
	Potassium (K$^+$) 3.0 mEq/L
	Calcium (Ca^{++}) 8.5 mg/dL
	SGOT (Serum glutanic-oxaloacetic transaminase)* 20 U/L
Hematology	Hemoglobin (Hbg) 11 g/dL
	Hematocrit (Hct) 50 percent (38–47)
	White blood cells (WBC) 9000 uL (mm^3)
	Red blood cells (RBC) 4.1 million μL (mm^3)
Coagulation	Prothrombin time (PT) 13 seconds

* Now called AST, aspartate aminotransferase.

LABORATORY VALUE ABBREVIATIONS

< = less than	mL = milliliter
> = more than	dL = deciliter
g = gram	U = unit
L = liter	mg = milligram
mEq = milliequivalent	µL = microliter

Bowel Hard, formed, brown stool. Stool specimen negative for occult blood.

Urine Amber colored, clear. Sp gr 1.025. Negative for leukocytes, nitrates, protein, glucose, ketones. Negative for WBCs, RBCs, and casts.

Diagnostic Studies

Chest x-ray	Clear lung fields
Electrocardiogram	Normal sinus rhythm (ECG)
Skin test	Positive allergens for grass
Mammogram	7/3/97
	Tumor 2 cm with no fixation to underlying pectoral fascia or muscle
Biopsy	7/3/97
	Left breast biopsy positive for primary tumor stage T1

■ TNM STAGING SYSTEM FOR BREAST CANCER—1992

I. Primary Tumor (T)
Definition: Classification of the primary tumor is the same for clinical and for pathologic classification.

TX Primary tumor cannot be assessed

T0 No evidence of primary tumor

Tis Carcinoma in situ: Intraductal carcinoma, lobular carcinoma in situ, or Paget's disease of the nipple with no tumor. (Paget's disease with a tumor is classified according to the size of the tumor.)

T1 Tumor 2.0 cm or less in greatest dimension
  T1a 0.5 cm or less
  T1b > 0.5 cm, but not > 1.0 cm
  T1c > 1.0 cm, but not > 2.0 cm

T2 Tumor > 2.0 cm, but not > 5.0 cm in greatest dimension

T3 Tumor > 5.0 cm in greatest dimension

T4 Tumor of any size with direct extension to chest wall or skin

T4a Extension to chest wall

T4b Edema (including peau d'orange) or ulceration of the skin of the breast or satellite skin nodules confined to the same breast

T4c Both T4a and T4b

T4d Inflammatory carcinoma (diffuse brawny induration of the skin of the breast with an erysipeloid edge, usually without an underlying palpable mass)

II. Regional Lymph Nodes (N)

NX Regional nodes cannot be assessed (eg, previously removed or no information on them can be obtained)

N0 No metastases

N1 Metastases in movable ipsilateral axillary lymph node(s)

N2 Metastases in ipsilateral axillary lymph node(s) fixed to each other or to other structures

N3 Metastases to ipsilateral internal mammary lymph node(s)

III. Pathologic Classification of Regional Lymph Nodes (pN)

pNx Cannot be assessed (previously removed, or not removed)

pN0 No metastases

pN1 Metastases to mobile ipsilateral axillary node(s)
  pN1a Only micrometastasis (ie, none > 0.2 cm)
  pN1b Metastasis with any > 0.2 cm)
    pN1bi Metastases in 1–3 nodes (all < 2.0 cm)
    pN1bii Metastases in 4 or more nodes (all < 2.0 cm)
    pN1biii Metastases < 2.0 cm with extension beyond the capsule of a lymph node
    pN1biv Metastases > 2.0 cm in diameter

pN2 Metastasis to ipsilateral axillary nodes fixed to one another or to other structures

pN3 Metastasis to ipsilateral internal mammary lymph node(s)

IV. Distant Metastasis (M)

MX Cannot be assessed

M0 None

M1 Distant metastasis present [includes metastasis to ipsilateral supraclavicular lymph node(s)]

Histopathologic Grade (G)

GX	Cannot be assessed
G1	Well differentiated
G2	Moderately differentiated
G3	Poorly differentiated
G4	Undifferentiated

TNM STAGE GROUPING—1992			
Stage 0	Tis	N0	M0
Stage I	T1	N0	M0
Stage IIA	T0	N1	M0
	T1	N1	M0
	T2	N0	M0
Stage IIB	T2	N1	M0
	T3	N0	M0

Stage IIIA	T0	N2	M0
	T1	N2	M0
	T2	N2	M0
	T3	N1	M0
	T3	N2	M0
Stage IIIB	T4	N (any)	M0
	T (any)	N3	M0
Stage IV	T (any)	N (any)	M1

Donegan & Spratt. *Cancer of the Breast* 4th ed. Philadelphia, PA: W. B. Saunders, 1995.

EXERCISE 9–A: *IDENTIFICATION OF SUBJECTIVE DATA*

The purpose of exercise 9–A is the identification of subjective data presented by the client in case study #2, Judith Smith. Fill in the blanks with subjective data noted in the case study. Examples of subjective data from case study #2 have been cited for each system.

Musculoskeletal

1. "I am tired at work lately."
2. "I fell in 1985 . . . and broke my left wrist and arm."
3.
4.
5.
6.
7.
8.

Cardiovascular

1. "My usual blood pressure is 120/80."
2.
3.

Gastrointestinal/Genitourinary

1. "I have a problem with constipation."
2.
3.

Integumentary/Food/Fluid

1. "I feel chilly."
2.
3.
4.
5.

Neurologic/Eye/Ear/Pain

1. "I wear glasses to read."
2. "I am having a migraine headache right now."
3. ___
4. ___
5. ___
6. ___
7. ___
8. ___

Respiratory

1. "I have hay fever."
2. ___
3. ___

Reproductive—female

1. "The doctor told me the tumor was malignant."
2. ___
3. ___
4. ___

Endocrine (None noted)

Psychiatric/Psychologic

1. "I am concerned about my radical mastectomy . . . tomorrow."
2. ___
3. ___
4. ___
5. ___
6. ___

Current Health Promotion Practices

1. "I shower each day."
2. "I drink 5 cups of coffee per day."
3. ___
4. ___
5. ___
6. ___
7. ___

Home Situation and Relationship With Others

1. "I wish my husband would hurry up and get here."
2. ___
3. ___
4. ___
5. ___

EXERCISE 9–B: *IDENTIFICATION OF OBJECTIVE DATA*

The purpose of Exercise 9–B is identification of objective data based on case study #2, Judith Smith. Fill in the blanks with the abnormal objective data from the case study. Examples of objective data from the case study are cited below for each system.

Musculoskeletal

1. Slight hand tremor.
2. Wrist 80–90 degree flexion and extension.
3.
4.
5.
6.
7.

Cardiovascular

1. Actual blood pressure 150/80 mm Hg.
2.
3.

Gastrointestinal/Genitourinary

1. Hard, formed, brown stool.
2.
3.

Integumentary/Food/Fluid

1. Skin warm to touch.
2.
3.
4.
5.

Neurologic/Eyes/Ears/Pain

1. Ability to read newsprint with glasses.
2. Grimacing.
3.
4.
5.
6.
7.
8.

Respiratory

1. Minimal wheezing on expiration.
2.
3.
4.

Reproductive—Female

1. Left breast biopsy positive primary tumor stage T1.
2.
3.
4.

Endocrine (None identified)

Psychiatric/Psychological

1. Facial muscles taut.
2.
3.
4.
5.
6.

Current Health Promotion Practices

1. Skin clean.
2. Drank 500–750 mg caffeine in coffee per day.
3.
4.
5.
6.

Home Situation and Relationship With Others

1. Husband not present.
2.
3.
4.
5.

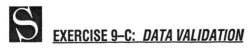

EXERCISE 9–C: *DATA VALIDATION*

The purpose of Exercise 9–C is to assist in comparing subjective and objective data to accepted normal values cited from the Judith Smith case study. Subjective data = SD; objective data = OD.

Musculoskeletal

1. Client value

SD: "I am tired at work lately."

OD: Slight hand tremor.

Normal value: No hand tremor.

2. Client value

SD: "I only sleep 2–3 hours."

OD: Dark circles under eyes.

Normal value:

3. Client value

SD: "My eyelids feel heavy."

OD: Ptosis.

Normal value:

4. Client value

SD: "I usually sleep 8 hours."

OD: Decreased attention span.

Normal value:

5. Client value

SD: "The doctor ordered sleeping medication for me."

OD: Temazepam 30 mg tab. 1 (PO) qhs prn ordered.

Normal value:

6. Client value

SD: "I am tired at work lately."

OD: Yawning during interview. Slouched posture.

Normal value:

7. Client value

SD: "I walk about 2 miles each evening."

OD: Firm muscle tone. No dyspnea upon exertion.

Normal value:

8. Client value

SD: "I fell in 1985 and broke my left wrist and arm."

OD: Wrist 80–90 degree flexion and extension.

Normal value:

Cardiovascular

1. Client value

SD: "My usual blood pressure is 120/80."

OD: Actual BP 150/80 mm Hg.

Normal value: 120/80 mm Hg.

2. Client value

SD: "My heart feels like it is racing."

OD: Apical rate 90 regular rhythm at rest.

Normal value:

3. Client value

SD: "My head has been pounding for the past 2 weeks."

OD: Rubbing forehead over left eye. BP 150/80; pulse 90.

Normal value:

Gastrointestinal/Genitourinary

1. Client value

SD: "I have a problem with constipation."

OD: Hard stool.

Normal value: Formed, moist stool.

2. Client value

SD: ". . . take Metamucil every night . . . Colace once a day."

OD: Abdomen moderately distended. Colace 100 mg/d prn.

Normal value:

3. Client value

SD: "I usually urinate six times a day."

OD: Specific gravity 1.025. Straw-colored, clear urine.

Normal value:

Integumentary

1. Client value

SD: "I feel chilly."

OD: Skin warm to touch.

Normal value: Skin warm to touch.

2. Client value

SD: "I feel nauseated and too upset to eat today."

OD: Ate 25% food on lunch tray.

Normal value:

3. Client value

SD: "I have lost 10 pounds in past 3 weeks."

OD: Actual weight 110 lb. Height 5′6″, small frame.

Normal value:

4. Client value

SD: "I eat 3 balanced meals a day."

OD: Typical daily intake not balanced with 4 food groups.

Normal value:

5. Client value

SD: "I drink 2 juice glasses of water a day."

OD: Skin turgor: shape returned in 10 seconds.

Normal value:

Neurologic/Eyes/Ears/Pain

1. Client value

SD: "I wear glasses at work to read fine print."

OD: Reads newsprint with glasses.

Normal value:

2. Client value

SD: ". . . Judith Smith. Monday, September 3, 1997 . . . at hospital . . . scheduled to have my breast removed . . . September 4, 1997."

OD: Oriented to time, place, person, and situation.

Normal value:

3. Client value

SD: ". . . migraine headaches for the past 20 years."

OD: Physician's note . . . treated migraine outpatient dept.

Normal value:

4. Client value

SD: "I am having a migraine headache right now."

OD: Grimacing.

Normal value:

5. Client value

SD: "It is steady throbbing pain around my left eye."

OD: Rubbing forehead over left eye. Lights off in room.

Normal value:

6. Client value

SD: "I rate the intensity a 7 on a scale of 0 to 10."

OD: Palpable neck and shoulder muscles.

Normal value:

7. Client value

SD: "I have no pain . . . in my left breast."

OD: Hard, irregular, poorly delineated, nonmobile lump.

Normal value:

8. Client value

SD: "I feel nauseated. . . ."

OD: Pale skin.

Normal value:

Respiratory

1. Client value

SD: "I wheeze when I get asthma."

OD: Minimal wheezing upon expiration.

Normal value:

2. Client value

SD: "I never smoked."

OD: Chest x-ray negative.

Normal value:

3. Client value

SD: "My eyes and nose have been itching. . . ."

OD: Nasal turbinates pale and edematous; lacrimation.

Normal value:

Reproductive-Female

1. Client value

SD: "The doctor told me the tumor was malignant."

OD: Breast biopsy positive for primary tumor stage T1.

Normal value:

2. Client value

SD: "I noticed the lump in my left breast. . . ."

OD: Demonstrated correct breast self-examination.

Normal value:

3. Client value

SD: "I have had a mammogram . . . annually for the past 11 years."

OD: Diagnostic studies reflect annual mammogram 1986–1997.

Normal value:

4. Client value

SD: "We use to have sex . . . once a week."

OD: Frown on face when discussing sexual relationship.

Normal value:

Endocrine (None identified)

Psychiatric/Psychological

1. Client value

SD: "I am concerned about my radical mastectomy tomorrow."

OD: Facial muscles taut.

Normal value:

2. Client value

SD: "I hope I can wear a bikini after this surgery."

OD: Speaking in a loud, abrupt voice. Eyes darting . . .

Normal value:

3. Client value

SD: "It is not fair."

OD: Eyes darting around room.

Normal value:

4. Client value

SD: "I believe that God is punishing me. . . ."

OD: Face flushed.

Normal value:

5. Client value

SD: "I told my husband . . . I would not go to church anymore."

OD: Constantly talking.

Normal value:

6. Client value

SD: "I rate my anxiety level a 2."

OD: Rated anxiety level a 2 on a scale of 0 to 5.

Normal value:

Current Health Promotion Practices

1. Client value

SD: "I shower and wash my hair every day." _____

OD: Skin clean. No body odor. _____

Normal value: Daily hygiene. _____

2. Client value

SD: "I scrub my teeth after every meal." _____

OD: 32 permanent teeth. No plaque. No dentures/plate. _____

Normal value: _____

3. Client value

SD: "I drink 5 cups of coffee per day." _____

OD: Drinks 500–750 mg caffeine per day. _____

Normal value: _____

4. Client value

SD: "I expect to be cured . . . after this surgery." _____

OD: Wringing hands. _____

Normal value: _____

5. Client value

SD: "My mother and grandmother died of breast cancer . . ." _____

OD: Carcinoma left breast, stage I. _____

Normal value: _____

6. Client value

SD: "My last [physical] exam was 2 months ago." _____

OD: Chart reflects yearly physical 1986–1994. _____

Normal value: _____

Home Situation and Relationship with Others

1. Client value

SD: "I wish my husband would hurry up and get here." _____

OD: Husband not present. _____

Normal value: _____

2. Client value

SD: "I am so nervous." _____

OD: Wringing hands. _____

Normal value: _____

3. Client value

SD: "I hope this surgery will not change my relationship with my husband."

OD: Began crying.

Normal value:

4. Client value

SD: "I love my husband and children."

OD: Smiled when talking about husband and children.

Normal value:

5. Client value

SD: At home, I go for walks just to get rid of all my anger."

OD: Began pacing floor. Wringing hands.

Normal value:

S EXERCISE 9–D: *IDENTIFICATION OF DYSFUNCTIONAL SYSTEMS*

The purpose of Exercise 9–D is to identify dysfunctional systems in the Judith Smith case study. Subjective and objective data were compared with normal values in Exercise 9–C. Based on the findings in Exercise 9–C, identify the systems that were dysfunctional, that is, the systems demonstrating a majority of abnormal values and standards. Mark (X) by YES or NO. YES indicates that the system is dysfunctional; NO means the system is not dysfunctional. As an exercise in critical thinking, write a statement to support your judgment for the answer you chose. Critical thinking establishes the logical reasoning for the selection of your responses. Citation of related literature may be required to support the rationale. An example is provided below for Musculoskeletal/Activity/Rest/Sleep.

Musculoskeletal/Activity/Rest/Sleep
Dysfunctional YES __X__   NO _____
Rationale: Slept 2–3 hours per night past 2 months. Change in sleep habit from optimal adult sleep pattern of 7–8 hours for age. Subjective data (verbal expression of fatigue) and objective data (dark circles under eyes) reflect sleep deprivation.

Cardiovascular
Dysfunctional YES _____   NO _____
Critical Thinking: _____

Gastrointestinal/Genitourinary
Dysfunctional YES _____   NO _____
Critical Thinking: _____

Integumentary
Dysfunctional   YES _____   NO _____
Critical Thinking: _____
_____
_____
_____
_____
_____

Neurologic/Eyes/Ears/Pain
Dysfunctional   YES _____   NO _____
Critical Thinking: _____
_____
_____
_____
_____
_____

Respiratory
Dysfunctional   YES _____   NO _____
Critical Thinking: _____
_____
_____
_____
_____
_____

Reproductive-female
Dysfunctional   YES _____   NO _____
Critical Thinking: _____
_____
_____
_____
_____
_____

Endocrine (none noted)

Psychiatric/Psychologic
Dysfunctional   YES _____   NO _____
Critical Thinking: _____
_____
_____
_____
_____
_____

Current Health Promotion Practices
Dysfunctional   YES _____   NO _____
Critical Thinking: _____
_____
_____
_____
_____

Home Situation and Relationships with Others

Dysfunctional YES _____ NO _____

Critical Thinking: _____

_____

_____

_____

_____

EXERCISE 9–E: *FORMULATING A THREE-PART NURSING DIAGNOSIS*

The purpose of Exercise 9–E is to illustrate the formulation of a three-part nursing diagnosis. The systems listed below were identified as dysfunctional in Exercise 9–D. For each dysfunctional system, formulate a minimum of one nursing diagnosis for Judith Smith. Refer to Appendix B for definitions of nursing diagnoses to determine the appropriate nursing diagnosis. An example of a nursing diagnosis is shown below for Musculoskeletal/Activity/Rest/Sleep.

Musculoskeletal/Activity/Rest/Sleep

1. Nursing diagnostic statement for dysfunctional system: Musculoskeletal/Activity/Rest/Sleep _____

   Nursing diagnostic label: Sleep-pattern disturbance _____

   Related to: Personal stress _____

   Defining characteristics (as evidenced by): Ptosis, dark circles under eyes, verbalized inability to sleep _____

2. Nursing diagnostic statement for dysfunctional system: Gastrointestinal/Genitourinary _____

   Nursing diagnostic label: _____

   Related to: _____

   Defining characteristics (as evidenced by): _____

   _____

   _____

   _____

3. Nursing diagnostic statement for dysfunctional system: Psychiatric/Psychologic _____

   Nursing diagnostic label: _____

   Related to: _____

   Defining characteristics (as evidenced by): _____

   _____

   _____

   _____

4. Nursing diagnostic statement for dysfunctional system: Integumentary/Food/Fluids _____

   Nursing diagnostic label: _____

   Related to: _____

   Defining characteristics (as evidenced by): _____

   _____

   _____

   _____

5. Nursing diagnostic statement for dysfunctional system: <u>Neurological/Eye/Ear/Pain</u>

   Nursing diagnostic label: _____

   Related to: _____

   Defining characteristics (as evidenced by): _____

   _____

   _____

   _____

6. Nursing diagnostic statement for dysfunctional system: <u>Respiratory</u>

   Nursing diagnostic label: _____

   Related to: _____

   Defining characteristics (as evidenced by): _____

   _____

   _____

   _____

7. Nursing diagnostic statement for dysfunctional system: <u>Reproductive-female</u>

   Nursing diagnostic label: _____

   Related to: _____

   Defining characteristics (as evidenced by): _____

   _____

   _____

   _____

8. Nursing diagnostic statement for dysfunctional system: <u>Current Health Promotion Practices</u>

   Nursing diagnostic label: _____

   Related to: _____

   Defining characteristics (as evidenced by): _____

   _____

   _____

   _____

9. Nursing diagnostic statement for dysfunctional system: <u>Home Situation and Relationship with Others</u>

   Nursing diagnostic label: _____

   Related to: _____

   Defining characteristics (as evidenced by): _____

   _____

   _____

   _____

EXERCISE 9–F: *RANKING NURSING DIAGNOSES*

The purpose of Exercise 9–F is to illustrate the ranking of nursing diagnoses in order of their priority—high, medium or low—with #1 the highest priority. Using Maslow's hierarchy of needs as the framework, rank the nursing diagnoses identified in Exercise 9–E, for Case Study #2. An example is provided below based on Exercise 9–E.

	NURSING DIAGNOSIS	MASLOW'S NEEDS	RANK
1.	Ineffective airway clearance	Physiologic	High
2.			
3.			
4.			
5.			
6.			
7.			
8.			
9.			

EXERCISE 9–G: *FORMULATING OUTCOME CRITERIA*

The purpose of Exercise 9–G is to illustrate formulation of outcomes for Judith Smith. Write outcome criteria for the four nursing diagnoses with the highest priority identified in Exercise 9–F. An example from case study #2 is cited below.

1. Nursing diagnosis: Ineffective airway clearance

   Outcome criteria

   Subject: Client

   Measurable verb: will deep-breathe and cough

   Outcome: using abdominal and accessory muscles

   Criteria: 5 min every 1 hour while awake

   Target time: by 9/5/97

2. Nursing diagnosis: _____

   Outcome criteria

   Subject: _____

   Measurable verb: _____

   Outcome: _____

   Criteria: _____

   Target time: _____

3. Nursing diagnosis: _____

   Outcome criteria

   Subject: _____

   Measurable verb: _____

   Outcome: _____

   Criteria: _____

   Target Time: _____

4. Nursing diagnosis: _____

   Outcome criteria

   Subject: _____

   Measurable verb: _____

   Outcome: _____

   Criteria: _____

   Target time: _____

 ### EXERCISE 9–H: WRITING NURSING INTERVENTIONS

The purpose of Exercise 9–H is to illustrate the writing of nursing interventions from outcomes. Using the outcomes listed in Exercise 9–G, write one nursing intervention for each outcome. An example from case study #2 is cited below.

1. Outcome criterion: <u>Client will deep-breathe and cough using abdominal and accessory muscles 5 minutes every 1 hour while awake by 9/5/97.</u>

   Nursing intervention
   _____

   Measurable verb: <u>explain and demonstrate</u>

   Subject: <u>client</u>

   Outcome: <u>therapeutic effects deep breathing and coughing q1h</u>

   Target time: <u>by 9/3/97</u>

   Signature: <u>Janet Jones, RN</u>

2. Outcome criterion: _____
   _____

   Nursing intervention

   Measurable verb: _____

   Subject: _____

   Outcome: _____

   Target time: _____

   Signature: _____

3. Outcome criterion: _____

_____

Nursing intervention

Measurable verb: _____

Subject: _____

Outcome: _____

Target time: _____

Signature: _____

4. Outcome criterion: _____

_____

Nursing intervention

Measurable verb: _____

Subject: _____

Outcome: _____

Target time: _____

Signature: _____

EXERCISE 9–I: WRITING A NURSING CARE PLAN FOR CASE STUDY #2, JUDITH SMITH

The purpose of Exercise 9–I is to illustrate the writing of a nursing care plan for case study #2. Using the following format, select one high-priority diagnosis from Exercise 9–F. Based on the nursing diagnosis that you chose, include the appropriate subjective data, objective data, body system, nursing diagnostic label, related to, and defining characteristics, nursing intervention, and the critical thinking to support each nursing intervention. Additional outcomes and nursing interventions may be written.

ASSESSMENT	NURSING DIAGNOSIS STATEMENT	OUTCOMES
Subjective Data Exercise 9–A, p. 131	*Nursing Label* _____	1: Subject: _____
_____	_____	Measurable Verb: _____
_____	*Related to* _____	Outcome: _____
_____	_____	Criterion: _____
_____	_____	Target Time: _____
Objective Data Exercise 9–B, p. 133	_____	2: Subject: _____
_____	_____	Measurable Verb: _____
_____	*Defining Characteristics (as evidenced by)*	Outcome: _____
_____	_____	Criterion: _____
DYSFUNCTIONAL BODY SYSTEM:	_____	Target Time: _____
_____	_____	
_____		

OUTCOMES (CONT)

3: Subject: _____

Measurable Verb: _____

Outcome: _____

Criterion: _____

Target Time: _____

NURSING INTERVENTIONS FOR

Outcome 1:
Measurable Verb: _____
Subject: _____
Outcome: _____
Target Time: _____
Signature: _____

Outcome 2:
Measurable Verb: _____
Subject: _____
Outcome: _____
Target Time: _____
Signature: _____

Outcome 3:
Measurable Verb: _____
Subject: _____
Outcome: _____
Target Time: _____
Signature: _____

CRITICAL THINKING FOR

Nursing Intervention
_____

Nursing Intervention
_____

Nursing Intervention
_____

EXERCISE 9–J: IDENTIFICATION OF INDEPENDENT NURSING

The purpose of Exercise 9–J is to identify independent nursing actions. Review the nursing interventions listed in Exercise 9–H, for case study #2. List below the nursing interventions that represent independent nursing actions. An example from case study #2 is provided below.

1. Teach client relaxation techniques. _____
2. _____
3. _____
4. _____
5. _____

EXERCISE 9–K: WRITING NURSES' NOTES

The purpose of Exercise 9–K is to illustrate writing accurate nurses' notes. Based on the following situation, write a Narrative, SOAP, and Focus nurse's note for the Judith Smith case study. Refer to examples for charting nurses' notes on pp. 66–68.

Situation for Exercise 9–K

Janet Jones, RN arrives in Mrs. Smith's room 9/3/97 at 1400, and the following scene and conversation ensues.

Mrs. Smith:	I am having a migraine headache. I feel nauseated. Please give me some medicine.
Nurse:	Where is your headache, and is the pain throbbing or sharp? How would you rate the pain on a scale on 0 to 10, with 0 no pain and 10 excruciating pain?
Mrs. Smith:	I rate my pain a 7. It feels like pressure over my left eye and causes my eye to tear.
Nurse:	What caused the headache to start?
Mrs. Smith:	I am so tense about this surgery. I take one ergotamine tablet when my headache begins. Aspirin does not help.
Nurse.	(Observes diaphoresis. Grimacing. Tearing left eye. Rubbing left forehead. Palpable neck and shoulder muscles. Lights off in room. Shades on window pulled. BP 146/80 lying. Apical pulse 90.)
Date 9/3/97	Time 1415
Nurse	(Administers ergotamine 2 mg sublingual tablet.)
Date 9/3/97	Time 1500
Nurse:	How would you rate your pain now, Mrs. Smith?
Mrs. Smith:	My migraine is a little better. I rate the pain a 4. My nausea is gone.
Nurse:	(Observes no grimacing. No diaphoresis. No rubbing left forehead). I plan to teach you distraction techniques to use when you feel another headache beginning.

S EXERCISE 9–K-1: WRITING *NARRATIVE* NURSES' NOTES

Date   Time   Nurse's Note

_____

S EXERCISE 9–K-2: WRITING *SOAP* NURSES' NOTES

Date   Time   Nurse's Note

S:

O:

A:

P:

S EXERCISE 9–K-3: WRITING *FOCUS* NURSES' NOTES

	Date	Time	Focus Nurse's Note

DATA:

_____

_____

_____

_____

_____

ACTION:

_____

_____

_____

_____

RESPONSE:

_____

_____

_____

TEACHING:

_____

_____

_____

_____

S EXERCISE 9–L: *EVALUATION OF OUTCOMES*

The purpose of Exercise 9–L is to evaluate the achievement of outcomes noted on the nursing care plan. In Exercise 9–G, outcomes were identified for case study #2. Based on the information related in the paragraph below, write an evaluation of whether the outcomes listed in Exercise 9–G were achieved.

Scene 9/13/97. Day of Surgery.

Mrs. Smith mastectomy was performed Thursday, 9/5/97. Upon returning to her hospital room, the nurse noticed that Mrs. Smith's children were present, but not Mr. Smith. Mrs. Smith stated, "My husband is on a business trip, and he will call me Sunday."

Scene 9/7/97. Discharge Date.

The nurse observed that Mrs. Smith had cried throughout her hospitalization. Her migraine headaches persisted after surgery with no relief from ergotamine. The nurse taught her how to rate her anxiety level on a scale of 1 to 5. "I rate my anxiety level a three." The nurse observed tht Mrs. Smith's incision was dry and intact. She verbalized no complaints of pain in the incisional area. Mrs. Smith stated, "I do not sleep at night. I tried relaxation exercises. I close my eyes, and try to visualize the sounds of the ocean." Dark circles and ptosis of eyelids present. Facial muscles taut. Verbalizes relaxation techniques. Nurse observed client practicing guided imagery intermittently. BP 150/80 sitting. Apical pulse 90. Lungs clear to auscultation. No edema nasal turbinates. No nasal drainage. No tearing eyes. Priest visited Mrs. Smith daily during her hospitalization. Continues to eat 25 percent of her meals. Demonstrated ability to bathe, feed, and dress self.

The nurse asked Mrs. Smith, "Will your husband take you home?" She stated, "He telephoned me today." Mrs. Smith's two children visited on the weekend, and informed the nurse that they will take their mother home, and contact their father.

1. Outcome criterion: <u>Explain and demonstrate to client therapeutic effects of deep breathing and coughing q1h by 9/3/97.</u>

   Resolved: YES __X__   NO _____

   Evaluation: <u>Client observed deep-breathing and coughing q1h postoperatively. Lungs clear to auscultation. No edema nasal turbinates. No nasal drainage. R 18.</u>

2. Outcome criterion: _____

   _____

   Resolved: YES _____   NO _____

   Evaluation: _____

   _____

   _____

3. Outcome criterion: _____

   _____

   Resolved: YES _____   NO _____

   Evaluation: _____

   _____

   _____

4. Outcome criterion: _____

   _____

   Resolved: YES _____   NO _____

   Evaluation: _____

   _____

   _____

 CORRECT RESPONSES FOR EXERCISES FOR CASE STUDY #2, JUDITH SMITH

EXERCISE 9–A: *IDENTIFICATION OF SUBJECTIVE DATA*

Musculoskeletal

1. "I am tired at work lately."
2. "I only sleep 2 to 3 hours."
3. "My eyelids feel heavy."
4. "I usually sleep 8 hours each night."
5. "The doctor ordered sleeping medication for me."
6. "I take a 15-minute rest when I arrive home from work."
7. "I walk about 2 miles a day."
8. "I fell . . . in 1985 and broke my left wrist and arm."

Cardiovascular

1. "My usual blood pressure is 120/80."
2. "My heart feels like it is racing."
3. "My head has been pounding for the past 2 weeks."

Gastrointestinal/Genitourinary

1. "I have a problem with constipation . . ."
2. ". . . take Metamucil every night . . . Colace once a day."
3. "I usually urinate six times a day."

Integumentary

1. "I feel chilly."
2. "I feel nauseated and too upset to eat today."
3. "I have lost 10 pounds in past 3 weeks."
4. "I usually eat three balanced meals a day."
5. ". . . drink two juice glasses of water a day."

Neurologic/Eyes/Ears/Pain

1. "I wear glasses to read."
2. "My name is Judith Smith . . . 9/3/97 . . . in Urban Hospital."
3. "I have had migraine headaches for the past 20 years."
4. "I am having a migraine headache right now."

5. "It is a steady, throbbing pain around my left eye."
6. "I rate the intensity a 7 on a scale of 0 to 10."
7. "I have no pain or tenderness in my left breast."
8. "I feel nauseated. . . ."

Respiratory

1. "I wheeze when I have an asthma attack."
2. "I never smoked."
3. "My eyes and nose have been itching. . . ."

Endocrine (None noted)

Reproductive-female

1. "The doctor told me the tumor was malignant."
2. "I noticed the lump in my left breast . . ."
3. "I have had a mammogram . . . every year for the past 5 years."
4. "We used to have . . . sex once a week."

Psychiatric/Psychologic

1. "I am concerned about my radical mastectomy . . . tomorrow."
2. "I hope I can wear a bikini . . ."
3. "This is not fair."
4. "I believe that God is punishing me . . ."
5. "I told my husband that I would not go to church . . ."
6. "I rate my anxiety level a 2."

Current Health Promotion Practices

1. "I shower each day."
2. "I scrub my teeth after every meal."
3. "I drink 5 cups of coffee every day."
4. "I expect to be cured of cancer after this surgery."
5. "My . . . grandmother . . . my mother died of breast cancer."
6. "I had my last [physical] exam 2 months ago."

Home Situation and Relationship With Others

1. "I wish my husband would hurry up and get here."
2. "I am so nervous."
3. "I hope this surgery will not change my relationship with my husband."
4. "I love my husband and children."
5. "At home, I go for walks just to get rid of my anger."

EXERCISE 9–B: *IDENTIFICATION OF OBJECTIVE DATA*

Musculoskeletal/Activity/Rest/Sleep

1. Slight hand tremor.
2. Dark circles under eyes.
3. Ptosis.
4. Decreased attention span.
5. Temazapam 30 mg Tab 1 (PO) qhs prn.
6. Yawning during interview. Slouched posture.
7. Firm muscle tone. No dyspnea upon exertion.
8. Wrist 80–90 degree flexion and extension.

Cardiovascular

1. Actual blood pressure 150/80 mm Hg.
2. Apical pulse rate 90.
3. Rubbing forehead over left eye. BP 150/80. P 90.

Gastrointestinal/Genitourinary

1. Hard, formed, brown-colored stool.
2. Abdomen moderately distended. Colace 100 mg/d.
3. Specific gravity 1.025. Urine straw-colored, clear.

Integumentary

1. Skin warm to touch.
2. Ate 25 percent food on lunch tray.
3. Actual weight 110 pounds. Height 5 feet 6 inches.
4. Daily 3 meals not balanced with basic 4 food groups.
5. Skin turgor: Shape returned in 10 seconds.

Neurologic/Eyes/Ears/Pain

1. Reads fine print with glasses.
2. Oriented to time, place, and person.
3. Physician noted 20-year history treatment migraine.
4. Grimacing.
5. Rubbing forehead over left eye.
6. Palpable neck and shoulder muscles.

Respiratory

1. Minimal wheezing on expiration.
2. Chest x-ray negative. No emphysema/SOB.
3. Nasal turbinates, pale, edematous; watery drainage.

Reproductive-female

1. Left breast biopsy positive primary tumor stage T1.
2. Demonstrated correct self-examination breast.
3. Diagnostic studies reflect yearly mammogram 1986–1997.
4. Frown on face when discussing sexual relationship.

Endocrine (None noted)

Psychiatric/Psychologic

1. Facial muscles taut.
2. Speaking in a loud, abrupt voice.
3. Eyes darting around room.
4. Face flushed.
5. Constantly talking.
6. BP 150/80. P 90. R 24.

Current Health Promotion Practices

1. Skin clean.
2. No plaque present. No dentures/plate. 32 permanent teeth.
3. Drinks 500–750 mg caffeine in coffee per day.
4. Wringing hands.
5. Genogram reflects family history breast cancer.
6. Chart reflects yearly physical 1986–1996.

Home Situation and Relationship With Others

1. Husband not present.
2. Wringing hands. Pacing floor.
3. Began crying.
4. Smiled when talking about husband and children.

EXERCISE 9–C: *DATA VALIDATION*

Musculoskeletal/Activity/Rest/Sleep

1. Client value

SD: "I am tired at work lately."

OD: Slight hand tremor.

Normal value: No hand tremor.

2. Client value

SD: "I sleep only 2 to 3 hours."

OD: Dark circles under eyes.

Normal value: No dark circles. 6–7 hours sleep/night.

3. Client value

SD: "My eyelids feel heavy."

OD: Ptosis.

Normal value: No ptosis.

4. Client value

SD: "I usually sleep 8 hours . . ."

OD: Decreased attention span.

Normal value: Ability to concentrate on task at hand.

5. Client value

SD: "The doctor ordered sleeping medication for me."

OD: Temazapam 30 mg Tab 1 (PO) qhs prn.

Normal value: Ability to sleep without sedatives.

6. Client value

SD: "I am tired at work lately."

OD: Yawning during interview. Slouched posture.

Normal value: No yawning. Posture erect.

7. Client value

SD: "I walk 2 miles each evening."

OD: Firm muscle tone. No dyspnea on exertion.

Normal value: Firm muscle tone. No dyspnea on exertion.

8. Client value

SD: "I fell . . . in 1985 and broke my left wrist and arm."

OD: Wrist 80–90 degree flexion and extension.

Normal value: Wrist 80–90 degree flexion and extension.

Cardiovascular

1. Client value

SD: "My usual blood pressure is 120/80."

OD: Actual BP 150/80 mm Hg.

Normal value: 120/80 mm Hg.

2. Client value

SD: "My heart feels like it is racing."

OD: Pulse rate 90 at rest.

Normal value: Average pulse for age 70–75.

3. Client value

SD: "My head has been pounding for the past 2 weeks."

OD: Rubbing forehead over left eye. BP 150/80. P 90.

Normal value: No pounding. BP 120/80. P 70–75.

Gastrointestinal/Genitourinary

1. Client value

SD: "I have a problem with constipation . . ."

OD: Hard, formed, brown stool.

Normal value: Formed, moist, brown stool.

2. Client value

SD: ". . . take Metamucil every night . . . take Colace once a day."

OD: Abdomen moderately distended. Colace 100 mg/qd PO prn.

Normal value: Regular bowel movements without laxatives.

3. Client value

SD: "I usually urinate six times a day."

OD: Specific gravity urine 1.025; straw-colored, clear.

Normal value: Sp gr. 1.003–1.030. Clear, straw-colored.

Integumentary

1. Client value

SD: "I feel chilly."

OD: Skin cool to touch.

Normal value: Skin warm to touch.

2. Client value

SD: "I feel nauseated and too upset to eat today."

OD: Ate 25 percent of food on lunch tray.

Normal value: Recommended amount nutrients consumed qd.

3. Client value

SD: "I have lost 10 pounds in 3 weeks."

OD: Actual weight 110 pounds; height 5′6″ . . . Small frame.

Normal value: 136–142 lb. average weight/5′6″/small frame.

4. Client value

SD: "I usually eat 3 balanced meals a day."

OD: Daily dietary intake lacked basic 4 food groups.

Normal value: Recommended amount nutrients consumed qd.

5. Client value

SD: "[I] drink two juice glasses of water a day."

OD: Skin turgor: shape returned in 10 seconds.

Normal value: 1200 mL intake qd. Immediate return skin.

Neurologic/Eyes/Ears/Pain

1. Client value

SD: "I wear glasses to read."

OD: Reads newsprint with glasses.

Normal value: Read newsprint without glasses.

2. Client value

SD: ". . . Judith Smith . . . September 3, 1997 . . . Urban Hospital . . . breast removal September 5, 1997."

OD: Oriented to time, place, person, and situation.

Normal value: Oriented to time, place, person, and situation.

3. Client value

SD: ". . . migraine headaches for the past 20 years."

OD: Physician's note stated 20-year treatment migraine.

Normal value: No migraine headaches.

4. Client value

SD: "I am having a migraine headache right now."

OD: Grimacing.

Normal value: No headaches.

5. Client value

SD: "It is a steady, throbbing pain around my left eye."

OD: Rubbing forehead over left eye. Lights off in room.

Normal value: No pain over left eye.

6. Client value

SD: "I rate the intensity a 7 on a scale of 0 to 10."

OD: Palpable neck and shoulder muscles.

Normal value: 0 intensity. Neck and shoulder muscles not palpable.

7. Client value

SD: "I have no pain or tenderness in my left breast."

OD: Hard, irregular, poorly delineated, nonmobile lump.

Normal value: Breast cancer painless; nontender 90% cases.

8. Client value

SD: ". . . I feel nauseated. . . ."

OD: Skin pale, perspiring.

Normal value: Pigmentation ranges from ivory to deep brown.

Respiratory

1. Client value

SD: "I wheeze when I have an asthma attack."

OD: Minimal wheezing on expiration.

Normal value: Lungs clear on auscultation. No allergies.

2. Client value

SD: "I never smoked."

OD: Chest x-ray negative. No emphysema/SOB.

Normal value: Chest x-ray negative; no emphysema; no SOB.

3. Client value

SD: "My eyes and nose have been itching. . . ."

OD: Nasal turbinates pale, edematous. Lacrimation.

Normal value: No edema nasal turbinates. No tearing eyes.

Reproductive-female

1. Client value

SD: "The doctor told me the tumor was malignant."

OD: Breast biopsy positive for primary tumor stage T1.

Normal value: No breast tumor. Negative biopsy results.

2. Client value

SD: "I noticed the lump . . . during my monthly self examination."

OD: Demonstrated correct breast self-examination.

Normal value: Monthly breast self-exam at regular time.

3. Client value

SD: "I have had a mammogram . . . annually for the past 11 years."

OD: Diagnostic studies reflect yearly mammogram 1986–1997.

Normal value: Yearly mammogram after age 50.

4. Client value

SD: "We used to have sex . . . once a week."

OD: Frown on face when discussing sexual relations.

Normal value: Cognitive knowledge about human sexuality.

Endocrine (None noted)

Psychiatric/Psychologic

1. Client value

SD: "I am concerned about my radical mastectomy . . . tomorrow."

OD: Facial muscles taut.

Normal value: Toned, not taut facial muscles.

2. Client value

SD: "I hope I can wear a bikini after this surgery."

OD: Speaking in loud abrupt tone. Constantly talking.

Normal value: Support system helps reduce stress level.

3. Client value

SD: "It is not fair."

OD: Eyes darting around room.

Normal value: Demonstrates effective coping skills.

4. Client value

SD: "I believe that God is punishing me for something."

OD: Face flushed. Facial muscles taut.

Normal value: Reality orientation to actual cause of problem.

5. Client value

SD: "I told my husband . . . I would not go to church anymore."

OD: Constantly talking.

Normal value: Problem solving. No transference of problem.

6. Client value

SD: "I rate my anxiety level a 2. . . ."

OD: Face flushed. Facial muscles taut. BP 150/80. P 90. R 24.

Normal value: Rates anxiety level 0. Free undue anxiety.

Current Health Promotion Practices

1. Client value

SD: "I shower . . . every day."

OD: Skin clean.

Normal value: Daily hygiene.

2. Client value

SD: "I scrub my teeth after every meal."

OD: 32 permanent teeth. No plaque. No dentures/plate.

Normal value: 32 permanent teeth. No plaque, dentures, plates.

3. Client value

SD: "I drink 5 cups of coffee per day. . . ."

OD: Drink 500–750 mg caffeine per day.

Normal value: 100–150 mg caffeine/qd; 100–150mg/c. coffee.

4. Client value

SD: "I expect to be cured . . . after this surgery."

OD: Wringing hands.

Normal value: Realistic expectations from surgery.

5. Client value

SD: "My maternal grandmother . . . and my mother died of breast cancer. . . ."

OD: Genogram reflects family history breast cancer.

Normal value: Presence risk factors predisposes to disease.

6. Client value

SD: ". . . my last [physical] exam was 2 months ago."

OD: Chart reflects yearly physical exams 1986–1997.

Normal value: Yearly examinations provide baseline data.

Home Situation and Relationships With Others

1. Client value

SD: "I wish my husband would hurry up and get here."

OD: Husband not present at admission interview.

Normal value: Significant other provides support system.

2. Client value

SD: "I am so nervous."

OD: Wringing hands. Pacing floor.

Normal value: Effective coping skills relieve anxiety.

3. Client value

SD: "I hope this surgery will not change my relationship with my husband."

OD: Began crying.

Normal value: Family assist in working through emotions.

4. Client value

SD: "I love my husband and children."

OD: Smiled when talking about husband and children.

Normal value: Seek and share love and belonging with others.

5. Client value

SD: "At home, I go for walks just to get rid of all my anger."

OD: Began pacing floor. Wringing hands.

Normal value: Effective coping skills relieve anxiety.

EXERCISE 9–D: *IDENTIFICATION OF DYSFUNCTIONAL SYSTEMS*

Musculoskeletal/Activity/Rest/Sleep
Dysfunctional   YES __X__   NO _____
Critical Thinking: Verbalized changes in sleeping habit from optimal adult sleep pattern of 7–8 hours for age. Slept 2–3 hours per night past 2 months. Subjective data (verbal expressions of fatigue) and objective data (dark circles under eyes) failed to meet accepted normal standards and values.

Cardiovascular
Dysfunctional   YES __X__   NO _____
Critical Thinking: Changes noted from client's baseline values and accepted normal values. Elevated blood pressure (150/80), increased pulse rate (90), and increased respirations (24). Verbalized sensation of head pounding. Values failed to meet accepted normal standards and values.

Gastrointestinal/Genitourinary
Dysfunctional   YES __X__   NO _____
Critical Thinking: Client verbalized changes in regularity of bowel elimination habits (constipation for the past 2 months). Insufficient roughage in diet. Stool softeners ineffective in remedying problem.

Integumentary
Dysfunctional   YES __X__   NO _____
Critical Thinking: Verbalized deviation from normal daily intake of food because of nausea. Weight 20 percent below ideal for height and frame. Weight loss indicated insufficient intake of nutrients to meet metabolic needs. Demonstrated decreased skin turgor with fluid intake less than normal 1200 mL/24 h.

Neurologic/Eyes/Ears/Pain
Dysfunctional   YES __X__   NO _____
Critical Thinking: Subjective data (nausea; rated pain a 7 on a scale of 0–10) and objective data (grimacing, rubbing forehead over left eye) provided evidence that the pain management was ineffective in alleviating the migraine headaches.

Respiratory
Dysfunctional   YES __X__   NO _____
Critical Thinking: History of hay fever and asthma. Inability to maintain clear airway at all times resulting from edema of nasal mucosa. Minimal wheezing sounds on expiration.

Reproductive-female
Dysfunctional   YES __X__   NO _____
Critical Thinking: Verbalized fear of husband's possible dissatisfaction with sexual relations as a result of mastectomy. Expressed perceived threat to sexual role. Inability of partners to discuss openly their feelings regarding the forthcoming mastectomy. No problem solving evident.

Psychiatric/Psychologic
Dysfunctional   YES __X__   NO _____
Critical Thinking: Verbalized increase in anxiety level (rated anxiety level a 2). Fear mastectomy will change her body image and relationship with husband. Ineffective individual and family coping skills demonstrated.

Current Health Promotion Practices
Dysfunctional   YES __X__   NO _____
Critical Thinking: Verbalized unrealistic expectations of surgery. Familial history of breast cancer. Intake of caffeine per day exceeded normal values (drank 500–750 mg caffeine in coffee per day). Excessive ingestion of caffeine may cause insomnia, restlessness, nausea, tachycardia.

Home Situation and Relationship With Others
Dysfunctional   YES __X__   NO _____
Critical Thinking: Proposed change in body image (mastectomy) caused a threat to client's self-concept and self-esteem. Husband not present. Lack of support from significant other increased client's anxiety level. Verbalized fear of mastectomy affecting relationship with husband. Lack of effective individual and family coping skills.

EXERCISE 9–E: *FORMULATING A NURSING DIAGNOSIS*

1. Nursing diagnosis

   Sleep-pattern disturbance related to personal stress as evidenced by ptosis, dark circles under eyes, verbalized inability to sleep.

2. Nursing diagnosis

   Constipation related to low-roughage diet and fluid intake as evidenced by hard, formed stools, use of laxatives, fluid intake less than normal 1200 mL/24 h.

3. Nursing diagnosis

   Body image disturbance related to perceived threat to self-concept as evidenced by verbalized increase in anxiety level, change in relationship with husband, fear of appearing less sexually attractive to husband.

4. Nursing diagnosis

   Fluid volume deficit related to deviation from normal fluid intake as evidenced by intake below normal 1200/qd, decreased skin turgor, Hct 50%.

5. Nursing diagnosis

   Pain related to physiologic injuring agent as evidenced by verbalized steady throbbing pain around left eye; rated pain 7 on a scale of 0–10; increased vital signs.

6. Nursing diagnosis

   Altered family processes related to situational crisis as evidenced by lack of support from husband, husband's inability to express feelings, client's verbal expressions of anxiety.

7. Nursing diagnosis

   Altered sexual patterns related to change in body function as evidenced by perceived threat to sexual role, fear of husband's dissatisfaction with client's body change, changes in husband's sexual behavior.

8. Nursing diagnosis

   Knowledge deficit therapeutic regimen related to misinterpretation of therapeutic interventions as evidenced by unrealistic expectations surgery results; excessive consumption of stimulant caffeine; unrealistic expectations of postoperative recovery period.

9. Nursing diagnosis

   Ineffective airway clearance related to excess thick secretions as evidenced by edematous nasal mucosa, nasal discharge, verbalized pruritus of eyes, tearing eyes, wheezing sounds on expiration, respirations 24; diaphoresis.

EXERCISE 9–F: *RANKING NURSING DIAGNOSES*

NURSING DIAGNOSES	MASLOW'S NEEDS	RANK
1. Ineffective airway clearance	Physiologic	High
2. Fluid volume deficit	Physiologic	High
3. Pain	Physiologic	High
4. Knowledge deficit	Safety	Medium
5. Altered family processes	Love/Belonging	Medium
6. Body image disturbance	Love/Belonging	Medium
7. Sleep pattern disturbance	Physiologic	Medium
8. Constipation	Physiologic	Medium
9. Altered sexual patterns	Love/Belonging	Low

EXERCISE 9–G: *FORMULATING OUTCOMES*

1. Outcome
   Subject: Client
   Measurable verb: will deep-breathe and cough
   Outcome: using abdominal and accessory muscles
   Criteria: 5 minutes every 1 hour while awake
   Target time: by 9/5/97

2. Outcome
   Subject: Client
   Measurable verb: will demonstrate
   Outcome: fluid and electrolyte balance
   Criteria: within normal limits
   Target Time: during the perioperative period

3. Outcome
   Subject: Client
   Measurable verb: will practice
   Outcome: guided imagery and rhythmic breathing
   Criteria: at onset of migraine q1h until migraine rated below 4
   Target time: 9/4/97

4. Outcome
   Subject: Client and husband
   Measurable verb: will describe
   Outcome: postoperative outcomes, possible complications, and discharge planning
   Criteria: realistically and accurately
   Target time: before scheduled surgery

EXERCISE 9–H: *WRITING NURSING INTERVENTIONS*

1. Nursing Intervention
   Measurable verb: <u>Explain and demonstrate</u>
   Subject: <u>to client</u>
   Outcome: <u>therapeutic effects deep-breathing and coughing q1h</u>
   Target time: <u>by 9/3/97</u>
   Signature: <u>Janet Jones, RN</u>

2. Nursing Intervention
   Measurable verb: <u>Monitor</u>
   Subject: <u>client's</u>
   Outcome: <u>intake & output; blood chemistry/ hematology values for compliance with normal values</u>
   Target time: <u>during perioperative period</u>
   Signature: <u>Janet Jones, RN</u>

3. Nursing Intervention
   Measurable verb: <u>Teach</u>
   Subject: <u>client</u>
   Outcome: <u>pain reduction through use of guided imagery</u>
   Target time: <u>by 9/4/97</u>
   Signature: <u>Janet Jones, RN</u>

4. Nursing Intervention
   Measurable verb: <u>Discuss</u>
   Subject: <u>with client and husband</u>
   Outcome: <u>pre/intra/postoperative care mastectomy client</u>
   Target time: <u>by 9/3/97</u>
   Signature: <u>Janet Jones, RN</u>

EXERCISE 9–I: CORRECT RESPONSE 1 TO WRITING A NURSING CARE PLAN FOR CASE STUDY #2, USING *FLUID VOLUME DEFICIT* AS THE HIGH-PRIORITY NURSING DIAGNOSIS

ASSESSMENT

Subjective Data
"I drink 2 juice glasses of water a day."
"I do not use diuretics."
"I am thirsty."

Objective Data
Skin turgor: shape returned in 10 seconds.
Hematocrit 50 percent
Intake below normal value of 1200 mL/d.

DYSFUNCTIONAL BODY SYSTEM
Cardiac

OUTCOME CRITERIA

1. Client will demonstrate fluid and electrolyte balance WNL during the perioperative period.

2. Client will verbalize factors leading to fluid volume deficit accurately by 9/4/97.

3. Client will verbalize the amount of fluid necessary to maintain fluid balance by 9/4/97.

NURSING DIAGNOSTIC STATEMENT

Nursing Diagnostic Label
Fluid volume deficit

Related to
deviation from normal fluid intake

Defining Characteristics (as evidenced by)
intake below normal 1200 mL/d, decreased skin turgor, Hct 50 percent

NURSING INTERVENTIONS

Outcome 1:
Monitor skin turgor, urine specific gravity, Hct, electrolytes, 24-hour intake and output by 9/3/97. Kathy Mayer, RN

Outcome 2:
Evaluate with client factors affecting fluid and electrolyte balance by 9/4/97. Kathy Mayer, RN

Outcome 3:
Teach the client normal fluid intake by 9/4/97. Kathy Mayer, RN

CRITICAL THINKING

Nursing Intervention
A balance of fluids and electrolytes is necessary for health and life. The balance of fluids and electrolytes in the body maintains physiologic homeostasis.

Nursing Intervention
Stress affects a client's fluid and electrolyte balance. The overall response of the body to stress is to increase the blood volume.

Nursing Intervention
The normal daily fluid intake is 2500 mL. The source of the intake is fluids, solid food, and water from oxidation. The normal output per day is 2500 mL.

EXERCISE 9–I: CORRECT RESPONSE 2 TO WRITING A NURSING CARE PLAN FOR CASE STUDY #2, USING *INEFFECTIVE AIRWAY CLEARANCE* AS THE HIGH-PRIORITY NURSING DIAGNOSIS

ASSESSMENT

Subjective Data
"I have hay fever."
"I wheeze when I have an asthma attack and get short of breath."
"My eyes and nose have been itching and watering this week."

Objective Data
Respirations 24; minimal wheezing on expiration both lungs; nasal mucosa pale and edematous.

DYSFUNCTIONAL BODY SYSTEM
Respiratory

NURSING DIAGNOSTIC STATEMENT

Nursing Label
Ineffective airway clearance

Related to
excess thick secretions

Defining Characteristics (as evidenced by)
nasal mucosa edematous, respirations 24, nasal drainage

OUTCOMES

1. Client will deep breath and cough using abdominal muscles 5 min q1h by 9/3/97.

2. Client will demonstrate use of nebulizer accurately by 9/5/97.

3. Client will verbalize effect of medications on breathing pattern by 9/5/97.

NURSING INTERVENTIONS

Outcome 1:
Teach client therapeutic effects of ventilating lungs today. Kathy Mayer, RN

Outcome 2:
Teach client to slow, deep-breathe with each whiff from nebulizer by 9/3/97. Kathy Mayer, RN

Outcome 3:
Instruct client to hold breath 10 sec when inhaling Alupent; wait 2 min between inhalations by 9/3/97. Kathy Mayer, RN

CRITICAL THINKING

Nursing Intervention
Deep breathing helps to remove mucus, aerate lung tissue, and prevent pneumonia.

Nursing Intervention
Deep breathing ensures maximum inflation of alveoli.

Nursing Intervention
Increased therapeutic effect of drug is achieved when administered properly.

(Continued)

ASSESSMENT

Subjective Data

Objective Data

DYSFUNCTIONAL BODY SYSTEM
Neurologic

OUTCOME CRITERIA

1. Client will verbalize pain rating before pain reaches a 4 by 9/4/97.

2. Client will practice guided imagery and rhythmic breathing at onset of migraine by 9/4/97.

3. Client will verbalize factors that trigger her migraine headaches by 9/4/97.

NURSING DIAGNOSIS

Nursing Diagnostic Label
Pain

Related to
physiologic injuring agent

Defining Characteristics (as evidenced by)
rated pain 7, grimacing, palpable neck and shoulder muscles

NURSING INTERVENTIONS

Outcome 1:
A: Teach client to rate pain on a scale of 0–10 by 9/3/97. Kathy Mayer, RN

Outcome 2:
B: Teach the client pain reduction through the use of guided imagery and rhythmic breathing by 9/4/97. Kathy Mayer, RN

Outcome 3:
C: Evaluate client's pain management plan by 9/3/97. Kathy Mayer, RN

CRITICAL THINKING

Nursing Intervention
The intensity or severity of pain is subjective. The pain rating scale is designed to assist the clients in describing the intensity of their pain.

Nursing Intervention
Relaxation techniques are effective in reducing stress, anxiety, muscle tension, and dissociation from pain.

Nursing Intervention
Identifying stress factors that trigger the migraine headaches will lead to the establishment of a realistic pain management program.

EXERCISE 9–J: *INDEPENDENT NURSING ACTIONS*

1. Teach client relaxation techniques.
2. Explain and demonstrate therapeutic effects of deep-breathing and coughing q1h.
3. Monitor intake and output; blood chemistry/ hematology values fall within normal values.
4. Teach client pain reduction through use guided imagery.

EXERCISE 9–K-1: *WRITING NARRATIVE NOTES*

Date 9/3/97   1400   Nurse's Note: Pain

"I am having a migraine headache. I feel nauseated. Please give me some medicine. I rate my pain a 7. It feels like pressure over my left eye and it causes my eye to tear. I am so tense about this surgery. Aspirin does not help. I take one ergotamine tablet when my headache begins." Diaphoretic. Facial grimacing. Tearing left eye. Rubbing left forehead. Palpable neck and shoulder muscles. Lights off in room; shade on window pulled. BP 146/80 lying. p 90. R 20.   —Janet Jones, RN

9/3/97   1415   Nurse's Note: Pain

Given ergotamine 2 mg sublingual. Taught distraction techniques.   —Janet Jones, RN

9/3/97   1500   Nurse's Note: Pain

"My migraine is a little better. I rate the pain a 4. My nausea is gone." No grimacing. No diaphoresis. No rubbing left forehead. Relief obtained from pain medication. Taught use guided imagery to alleviate pain.   —Janet Jones, RN

EXERCISE 9–K-2: *WRITING SOAP NURSES' NOTES*

Date 9/3/97   Time 1400   Nurse's Note: Pain

S: "I am having a migraine headache. I feel nauseated. Please give me some medicine. I rate my pain a 7. It feels like pressure over my left eye and causes my eye to tear. I am so tense about this surgery. Aspirin does not help. I take ergotamine one tablet when my headache begins. "

O: Diaphoretic. Grimacing. Tearing left eye. Rubbing left forehead. Palpable neck and shoulder muscles. Lights off in room shades on window pulled. BP 146/80 lying. P 90. R 20.

A: No relief from migraine. Pain persists.

P: Administer pain medication. Teach distraction techniques.   —Janet Jones, RN

Date 9/4/97   Time 1415   Nurse's Note: Pain

I: Ergotamine 2mg sublingual given. Taught distraction techniques for relaxation.

                              —Janet Jones, RN

Date 9/4/97   Time 1500   Nurse's Note: Pain

E: "My migraine is a little better. I rate the pain a 4. My nausea is gone."

No grimacing. No diaphoresis. No rubbing left forehead. Relief obtained from pain medication.

R: Teach use guided imagery to alleviate pain.
                              —Janet Jones, RN

EXERCISE 9–K-3: *WRITING FOCUS NURSES' NOTES*

Date 9/3/97   Time 1400   FOCUS Nurse's Note: Pain

DATA: 'I am having a migraine headache. I feel nauseated. Please give me some medicine. I rate my pain a 7. It feels like pressure over my left eye and causes my eye to tear. I am so tense about this surgery. Aspirin does not help. I take one ergotamine tablet when my headache begins." Diaphoretic. Grimacing. Tearing left eye. Rubbing left forehead. Palpable neck and shoulder muscles. Lights off in room. Shades on window pulled. BP 146/80 lying. P 90. R 20.   —Janet Jones, RN

9/3/97   1415   FOCUS Nurse's Note: Pain

ACTION: Ergotamine 2 mg sublingual given. Taught distraction techniques.

                              —Janet Jones, RN

9/3/96   1500   FOCUS Nurse's Note: Pain

RESPONSE: "My migraine is a little better. I rate the pain a 4. My nausea is gone." No grimacing. No diaphoresis. No rubbing left forehead. Relief obtained from pain medication.

TEACHING: Taught use guided imagery to alleviate pain.   —Janet Jones, RN

EXERCISE 9–L: *EVALUATION OF THE ACHIEVEMENT OF OUTCOMES*

1. Outcome: <u>Explain and demonstrate to client the therapeutic effects of deep breathing and coughing q1h 9/3/97.</u>

   Resolved: YES <u> X </u>   NO <u>____</u>

   Evaluation: <u>Client observed deep breathing and coughing q1h postoperatively. Lungs clear to auscultation. No edema nasal turbinates. No nasal drainage. R 18.</u>

2. Outcome: <u>Monitor client's intake and output; blood chemistry/hematology values fall within normal values.</u>

   Resolved: YES <u> X </u>   NO <u>____</u>

   Evaluation: <u>Fluid and electrolytes and hematology values within normal limits by surgery 9/4/97, and within normal limits at discharge.</u>

3. Outcome: <u>Client will practice guided imagery at onset migraine and q1h until migraine pain is rated below a 4.</u>

   Resolved: YES <u>____</u>   NO <u> X </u>

   Evaluation: <u>Client practiced guided imagery sporadically during the postoperative period. Husband not present during the preoperative and intraoperative periods. Husband present postoperatively. Husband and wife taught imagery. Client continues practicing imagery sporadically.</u>

4. Outcome: <u>Client and husband will describe postoperative outcomes, possible complications, and discharge planning realistically and accurately before scheduled surgery.</u>

   Resolved: YES <u>____</u>   NO <u> X </u>

   Evaluation: <u>Surgeon discussed postoperative outcomes and possible complications with client. Husband not present pre/intraoperatively. Discharge planning discussed with client postoperatively. Client demonstrates unrealistic expectations of self and plans to return to work in 2 weeks.</u>

Appendices

Appendix A
NANDA Taxonomy I, Revised 1994

PATTERN 1: EXCHANGING

1.1.2.1.	Altered nutrition: more than body requirements
1.1.2.2.	Altered nutrition: less than body requirements
1.1.2.3.	Altered nutrition: potential for more than body requirements
1.2.1.1.	Risk for infection
1.2.2.1.	Risk for altered body temperature
1.2.2.2.	Hypothermia
1.2.2.3.	Hyperthermia
1.2.2.4.	Ineffective thermoregulation
1.2.3.1.	Dysreflexia
1.3.1.1.	Constipation
1.3.1.1.1.	Perceived constipation
1.3.1.1.2.	Colonic constipation
1.3.1.2.	Diarrhea
1.3.1.3.	Bowel incontinence
1.3.2.	Altered urinary elimination
1.3.2.1.1.	Stress incontinence
1.3.2.1.2.	Reflex incontinence
1.3.2.1.3.	Urge incontinence
1.3.2.1.4.	Functional incontinence
1.3.2.1.5.	Total incontinence
1.3.2.2.	Urinary retention
1.4.1.1.	Altered (specify type) tissue perfusion (Renal, cerebral, cardiopulmonary, gastrointestinal, peripheral)
1.4.1.2.1.	Fluid volume excess
1.4.1.2.2.1.	Fluid volume deficit
1.4.1.2.2.2.	Potential fluid volume deficit
1.4.2.1.	Decreased cardiac output
1.5.1.1.	Impaired gas exchange
1.5.1.2.	Ineffective airway clearance
1.5.1.3.	Ineffective breathing pattern
1.5.1.3.1.	Inability to sustain spontaneous ventilation
1.5.1.3.2.	Dysfunctional ventilatory weaning response (DVWR)
1.6.1.	Risk for injury
1.6.1.1.	Risk for suffocation
1.6.1.2.	Risk for poisoning
1.6.1.3.	Risk for trauma
1.6.1.4.	Risk for aspiration
1.6.1.5.	Risk for disuse syndrome
1.6.2.	Altered protection
1.6.2.1.	Impaired tissue integrity
1.6.2.1.1.	Altered oral mucous membrane
1.6.2.1.2.1.	Impaired skin integrity
1.6.2.1.2.2.	Risk for impaired skin integrity

PATTERN 2: COMMUNICATING

2.1.1.1.	Impaired verbal communication

PATTERN 3: RELATING

3.1.1.	Impaired social interaction
3.1.2.	Social isolation
3.1.3.	Risk for loneliness
3.2.1.	Altered role performance
3.2.1.1.1.	Altered parenting
3.2.1.1.2.	Risk for altered parenting
3.2.1.1.2.1.	Risk for altered parent/infant/child attachment
3.2.1.2.1.	Sexual dysfunction
3.2.2.	Altered family processes
3.2.2.1.	Caregiver role strain
3.2.2.3.1.	Altered family process: alcoholism

3.2.3.1.	Parental role conflict
3.3.	Altered sexuality patterns

PATTERN 4: VALUING

4.1.1.	Spiritual distress (distress of the human spirit)
4.2.	Potential or enhanced spiritual well-being

PATTERN 5: CHOOSING

5.1.1.1.	Ineffective individual coping
5.1.1.1.1.	Impaired adjustment
5.1.1.1.2.	Defensive coping
5.1.1.1.3.	Ineffective denial
5.1.2.1.1.	Ineffective family coping: disabling
5.1.2.1.2.	Ineffective family coping: compromised
5.1.2.2.	Family coping: potential for growth
5.1.3.1.	Potential for enhanced community coping
5.1.3.2.	Ineffective community coping
5.2.1.1.	Noncompliance (specify)
5.2.2.	Ineffective management of therapeutic regimen: families
5.2.3.	Ineffective management of therapeutic regimen: community
5.2.4.	Ineffective management of therapeutic regimen: individual
5.3.1.1.	Decisional conflict (specify)
5.4.	Health-seeking behaviors (specify)

PATTERN 6: MOVING

6.1.1.1.	Impaired physical mobility
6.1.1.1.1.	Risk for peripheral neurovascular dysfunction
6.1.1.1.2.	Risk for perioperative positioning injury
6.1.1.2.	Activity intolerance
6.1.1.2.1.	Fatigue
6.1.1.3.	Risk for activity intolerance
6.2.1.	Sleep pattern disturbance
6.3.1.1.	Diversional activity deficit
6.4.1.1.	Impaired home maintenance management
6.4.2.	Altered health maintenance
6.5.1.	Feeding self-care deficit
6.5.1.1.	Impaired swallowing
6.5.1.2.	Ineffective breast-feeding
6.5.1.2.1.	Interrupted breast-feeding
6.5.1.3.	Effective breast-feeding
6.5.1.4.	Ineffective infant feeding pattern

6.5.2.	Bathing/hygiene self-care deficit
6.5.3.	Dressing/grooming self-care deficit
6.5.4.	Toileting self-care deficit
6.6.	Altered growth and development
6.7.	Relocation stress syndrome
6.8.1.	Risk for disorganized infant behavior
6.8.2.	Disorganized infant behavior
6.8.3.	Potential for enhanced organized infant behavior

PATTERN 7: PERCEIVING

7.1.1.	Body image disturbance
7.1.2.	Self-esteem disturbance
7.1.2.1.	Chronic low self-esteem
7.1.2.2.	Situational low self-esteem
7.1.3.	Personal identity disturbance
7.2.	Sensory/perceptual alterations (specify: visual, auditory, kinesthetic, gustatory, tactile, olfactory)
7.2.1.1.	Unilateral neglect
7.3.1.	Hopelessness
7.3.2.	Powerlessness

PATTERN 8: KNOWING

8.1.1.	Knowledge deficit (specify)
8.2.1.	Impaired environmental interpretation syndrome
8.2.2.	Acute confusion
8.2.3.	Chronic confusion
8.3.	Altered thought processes
8.3.1.	Impaired memory
8.3.	Altered thought processes

PATTERN 9: FEELING

9.1.1.	Pain
9.1.1.1.	Chronic pain
9.2.1.1.	Dysfunctional grieving
9.2.1.2.	Anticipatory grieving
9.2.2.	Risk for violence: self-directed or directed at others
9.2.2.1.	Risk for self-mutilation
9.2.3.	Post-trauma response
9.2.3.1.	Rape-trauma syndrome
9.2.3.1.1.	Rape-trauma syndrome: compound reaction
9.2.3.1.2.	Rape-trauma syndrome: silent reaction
9.3.1.	Anxiety
9.3.2.	Fear

Appendix B
NANDA's 1994 List of Approved Nursing Diagnoses, Definitions, Related Factors, and Defining Characteristics

The following list represents the NANDA-approved nursing diagnoses for clinical use and testing (1994). The list is not final and requires continual research. Square brackets indicate material added by the author.

ACTIVITY INTOLERANCE

Definition: A state in which an individual has insufficient physiologic or psychologic energy to endure or complete required or desired daily activities.

Related factors: Bed rest; immobility; generalized weakness; sedentary life-style; imbalance between oxygen supply and demand.

Defining characteristics: Verbal report of fatigue or weakness; abnormal heart rate or blood pressure response to activity, exertional discomfort, or dyspnea; electrocardiographic changes reflecting arrhythmias or ischemia.

ACTIVITY INTOLERANCE, RISK FOR

Definition: A state in which an individual is at risk of experiencing insufficient physiologic or psychologic energy to complete required or desired daily activities.

Related to the presence of risk factors: History of previous intolerance; [sedentary life-style]; deconditioned status; presence of circulatory or respiratory problems; inexperience with the activity.

NUTRITION: LESS THAN BODY REQUIREMENTS, ALTERED

Definition: An individual experiences an intake of nutrients insufficient to meet metabolic needs.

Related factors: Inability to ingest or digest food or absorb nutrients due to biologic, psychologic, or economic factors.

Defining characteristics: Loss of weight with adequate food intake; body weight 20 percent or more below ideal for height and frame; reported food intake less than recommended daily allowance (RDA); reported weakness of muscles required for swallowing or mastication; reported altered taste sensation; satiety immediately after ingesting food; abdominal pain with or without pathology; sore, inflamed buccal cavity; capillary fragility; abdominal cramping; diarrhea or steatorrhea; hyperactive bowel sounds; lack of interest in food; perceived ability to ingest food; pale conjunctival and mucous membranes; poor muscle tone; excessive loss of hair; lack of information, misinformation, misconceptions.

NUTRITION: MORE THAN BODY REQUIREMENTS, ALTERED

Definition: An individual experiences an intake of nutrients that exceeds metabolic needs.

Related factors: Excessive intake in relation to metabolic need.

Defining characteristics: Weight 20 percent over ideal for height and frame; triceps skin fold greater than 15 mm in men, 25 mm in women; sedentary activity level; reported or observed dysfunctional eating pattern: pairing food with other activities; concentrating food intake at the end of day; eating in response to external cues such as time of day, social situation; eating in response to internal cues other than hunger anxiety; [viewing food as a reward].

NUTRITION: POTENTIAL FOR MORE THAN BODY REQUIREMENTS, ALTERED

Definition: An individual is at risk for experiencing an intake of nutrients that exceeds metabolic needs.

Related to the presence of risk factors: Reported or observed obesity in one or both parents; rapid transition across growth percentiles in infants or children; reported use of solid food as major food source before 5 months of age; observed use of food as reward or comfort measure; reported or observed higher baseline weight at beginning of each pregnancy; dysfunctional eating patterns: pairing food with other activities; concentrating food intake at end of day; eating in response to external cues such as the time of day; eating in response to internal cues other than hunger (anxiety).

INFECTION, RISK FOR

Definition: An individual is at increased risk for invasion by pathogenic organisms.

Related to the presence of risk factors: Inadequate primary defenses, e.g., broken skin, traumatized tissue, decrease in ciliary action, stasis of body fluids, change in pH secretions, altered peristalsis; inadequate secondary defense, for example, decreased hemoglobin, leukopenia, suppressed inflammatory response and immunosuppression; inadequate acquired immunity; tissue destruction and increased environmental exposure; chronic disease; invasive procedures; malnutrition; trauma; lack of knowledge to avoid exposure to pathogens; pharmaceutic agents.

TEMPERATURE, RISK FOR ALTERED BODY

Definition: The individual is at risk for failure to maintain body temperature within normal range.

Related to the presence of risk factors: Extremes of age; extremes of weight; exposure to extremes in environmental temperature; inactivity or vigorous activity; altered metabolic rate; sedation; inappropriate clothing for environmental temperature; dehydration; illness or trauma affecting temperature regulation.

HYPOTHERMIA

Definition: An individual's body temperature is reduced below normal range.

Related factors: Damage to hypothalamus; exposure to cool or cold environment; inability or decreased ability to shiver; malnutrition; inadequate clothing; consumption of alcohol; medications causing vasodilation; evaporation from cool environment; decreased metabolic rate, inactivity; aging.

Defining characteristics: Reduction in body temperature below normal range; shivering; cool skin; pallor.

HYPERTHERMIA

Definition: An individual's body temperature is elevated above his/her normal range.

Related factors: Exposure to hot environment; increased metabolic rate; dehydration; medications; anesthesia; inappropriate clothing; decreased ability to perspire; illness or trauma.

Defining characteristics: Increase in body temperature above normal range; flushed skin; warm to touch; increased respiratory rate; tachycardia; convulsions.

THERMOREGULATION, INEFFECTIVE

Definition: The individual's temperature fluctuates between hypothermia and hyperthermia.

Related factors: Trauma or illness; immaturity; aging; fluctuating environmental temperature.

Defining characteristics: Fluctuation in body temperature above or below the normal range. See characteristics present in hypothermia and hyperthermia.

DYSREFLEXIA

Definition: An individual with a spinal cord injury at T7 or above experiences a life-threatening, uninhibited sympathetic response of the nervous system to a noxious stimulus.

Related factors: Bladder distention; bowel distention; skin irritation; lack of patient and caregiver knowledge.

Defining characteristics:
Major: Paroxysmal hypertension (sudden periodic elevated blood pressure where systolic pressure is over 140 mm Hg and diastolic is above 90 mm Hg); bradycardia or tachycardia (pulse rate of less than 60 or over 100 beats per minute); diaphoresis (above the injury); red splotches on skin (above the injury); pallor (below the injury); headache (a diffuse pain in different portions of the head and not confined to any nerve distribution area).
Minor: Chilling; conjunctival congestion; Horner's syndrome (contraction of the pupil, partial ptosis, enophthalmos, and sometimes loss of sweating over the affected side of the face); paresthesia; pilomotor reflex; blurred vision; chest pain; metallic taste in mouth; nasal congestion.

CONSTIPATION

Definition: An individual experiences a change in normal bowel habits characterized by a decrease in frequency and/or passage of hard, dry stools.

Related factors: Low-roughage diet, low-fluid intake, decreased activity level, absence of routine time for bowel movements, side effect of medications.

Defining characteristics: Decreased activity level; frequency of stool less than usual pattern; hard, formed stools; palpable mass; reported feeling of pressure in rectum; straining at stool; [decreased bowel sounds; abdominal distention].

CONSTIPATION, PERCEIVED

Definition: An individual makes a self-diagnosis of constipation and ensures a daily bowel movement through abuse of laxatives, enemas, and suppositories.

Related factors: Cultural and family health beliefs; faculty appraisal; impaired thought processes.

Defining characteristics: Expectation of a daily movement, with the resulting overuse of laxatives, enemas, and suppositories; expected passage of stool at same time every day.

CONSTIPATION, COLONIC

Definition: An individual's pattern of elimination is characterized by hard, dry stool that results from a delay in passage of food residue.

Related factors: Less than adequate fluid intake; less than adequate dietary intake; less than adequate fiber; less than adequate physical activity; immobility; lack of privacy; emotional disturbances; chronic use of medication and enemas; stress; change in daily routine; metabolic problems (hypothyroidism, hypocalcemia, hypokalemia).

Defining characteristics: Decreased frequency; hard, dry stool; straining at stool; painful defecation; abdominal distention; palpable mass.

DIARRHEA

Definition: An individual experiences a change in normal bowel habits characterized by the frequent passage of loose, fluid, unformed stools.

Related factors: Gastrointestinal disorders; metabolic disorders; nutritional disorders; endocrine disorders; infectious processes; tube feedings; fecal impaction; change in dietary intake; adverse affects of medications; high-stress levels; [food intolerance; medications; stress; contaminants; tube feedings].

Defining characteristics: Abdominal pain; cramping, increased frequency; increased frequency of bowel sounds; loose, liquid stools; urgency

BOWEL INCONTINENCE

Definition: An individual experiences a change in normal bowel habits characterized by involuntary passage of stool.

Related factors: Gastrointestinal disorders; neuromuscular disorders; colostomy; loss of rectal sphincter control; impaired cognition; [decreased level of consciousness; poor sphincter control].

Defining characteristics: Involuntary passage of stool.

URINARY ELIMINATION, ALTERED

Definition: An individual experiences a disturbance in urine elimination.

Related factors: Multiple causality, including: anatomic obstruction, sensory motor impairment, urinary tract infection.

Defining characteristics: Dysuria; frequency; hesitancy; incontinence; nocturia; retention; urgency.

INCONTINENCE, STRESS

Definition: The state in which an individual experiences a loss of urine of less than 50 mL occurring with increased abdominal pressure.

Related factors: Degenerative changes in pelvic muscles and structural supports with increased age: high intra-abdominal pressures, e.g., obesity; gravid uterus; incompetent bladder outlet; overdistention between voiding; weak pelvic muscles and structural supports.

Defining characteristics: Reported or observed dribbling with increased abdominal pressure; urinary urgency; urinary frequency, e.g., more often than every 2 hours.

INCONTINENCE, REFLEX

Definition: The state in which an individual experiences an involuntary loss of urine, occurring at somewhat predictable intervals when a specific bladder volume is reached.

Related factors: Neurologic impairment, e.g., spinal cord lesion that interferes with conduction of cerebral messages above the level of the reflex arc.

Defining characteristics: No awareness of bladder filling; no urge to void or feelings of bladder fullness; uninhabited bladder contraction or spasm at regular intervals.

INCONTINENCE, URGE

Definition: The state in which an individual experiences involuntary passage of urine occurring soon after a strong sense of urgency to void.

Related factors: Decreased bladder capacity; irritation of bladder stretch receptors causing spasm, e.g., bladder infection; alcohol; caffeine; increased fluids; increased urine concentration; overdistention of bladder.

Defining characteristics: Urinary urgency; frequency (e.g., voiding more often than every 2 hours); bladder contracture or spasms.

INCONTINENCE, FUNCTIONAL

Definition: The state in which an individual experiences an involuntary, unpredictable passage of urine.

Related factors: Altered environment; sensory, cognitive, or mobility deficits.

Defining characteristics: Urge to void or bladder contractions sufficiently strong to result in loss of urine before reaching an appropriate receptacle.

INCONTINENCE, TOTAL

Definition: The state in which an individual experiences a continuous and unpredictable loss of urine.

Related factors: Neuropathy preventing transmission of reflex indicating bladder fullness; neurologic dysfunction causing triggering of micturition at unpredictable times; independent contraction of detrusor reflex resulting from surgery; trauma or disease affecting spinal cord nerves; anatomic, e.g., fistula.

Defining characteristics: Constant flow of urine occurs at unpredictable times without distention or uninhibited bladder contraction or spasms; unsuccessful incontinence refractory treatments; nocturia.

URINARY RETENTION

Definition: The individual experiences incomplete emptying of the bladder.

Related factors: High urethral pressure caused by weak detrusor; inhibition of reflex arc; strong sphincter; blockage.

Defining characteristics: Bladder distention; small, frequent voiding or absence of urine output.

TISSUE PERFUSION ALTERED (specify type: renal, cerebral, cardiopulmonary, gastrointestinal, or peripheral).

Definition: An individual experiences a decrease in nutrition and oxygenation at the cellular level resulting from a deficit in capillary blood supply.

Related factors: Interruption of flow, arterial; interruption of flow, venous; exchange problems; hypovolemia; hypervolemia.

Defining characteristics: Cold extremities; dependent blue or purple skin color; pale on elevation—color does not return on lowering of leg; diminished arterial pulsations; shining skin; lack of lanugo; slow-growing, dry brittle nails; claudication; bruits; slow healing of lesions.

FLUID VOLUME EXCESS

Definition: An individual experiences increased fluid retention and edema.

Related factors: Compromised regulatory mechanism; excess fluid intake; excess sodium intake.

Defining characteristics: Edema; effusion; anasarca; weight gain; shortness of breath; orthopnea; intake greater than output; S3 heart sound; pulmonary congestion (as seen on chest x-ray); abnormal breath sounds, rales (crackles); decreased hemoglobin and hematocrit; change in respiratory pattern; change in mental status; blood pressure changes; central venous pressure changes; pulmonary artery pressure changes; jugular vein distention; positive hepatojugular reflex; oliguria; changes in specific gravity; azotemia; altered electrolytes; restlessness and anxiety.

FLUID VOLUME DEFICIT

Definition: The state in which an individual experiences vascular, cellular, or intracellular dehydration.

Related factors: Active fluid volume loss; failure of regulatory mechanisms.

Defining characteristics: Change in urine output; change in urine concentration; sudden weight loss or gain; decreased venous filling; hemoconcentration; change in serum sodium.

FLUID VOLUME DEFICIT, RISK FOR

Definition: The state in which an individual is at risk for experiencing vascular, cellular, or intracellular dehydration.

Related to the presence of risk factors: Extremes of age [infant; elderly]; lack of access to fluids; knowledge deficit related to fluid volume; medications (e.g., diuretics); immobility; hypermetabolic state; excessive losses through normal routes (e.g., diarrhea); excessive losses through abnormal routes (e.g., indwelling tubes); failure to drink sufficient amounts fluid.

DECREASED CARDIAC OUTPUT

Definition: A state in which the blood pumped by an individual's heart is sufficiently reduced that it is inadequate to meet the needs of the body's tissues.

Related factors: Side effects of medications, e.g., cocaine, effect alcohol on the heart muscle, electrical alteration in rate, rhythm, conduction.

Defining characteristics: Variations in blood pressure readings; arrhythmias; fatigue; jugular vein distention; color changes, skin and mucous membranes; oliguria; decreased peripheral pulses; cold, clammy skin; adventitious breath sounds (crackles); dyspnea; orthopnea; restlessness.

IMPAIRED GAS EXCHANGE

Definition: The state in which the individual experiences a decreased passage of oxygen and/or carbon dioxide between the alveoli of the lungs and the vascular system.

Related factors: Ventilation-perfusion imbalance.

Defining characteristics: Confusion; somnolence; restlessness; irritability; inability to move secretions; hypercapnia; hypoxia.

INEFFECTIVE AIRWAY CLEARANCE

Definition: A state in which an individual is unable to clear secretions or obstructions from the respiratory tract to maintain airway patency.

Related factors: Decreased energy and fatigue; tracheobronchial infection; obstruction; excess thick secretions; perceptual-cognitive impairment; trauma.

Defining characteristics: Abnormal breath sounds: rales (crackles), rhonchi (wheezes); changes in rate or depth of respiration; tachypnea; cough, effective or ineffective, with or without sputum; cyanosis; dyspnea.

INEFFECTIVE BREATHING PATTERN

Definition: The state in which an individual's inhalation and or exhalation pattern does not enable adequate pulmonary inflation or emptying.

Related factors: Neuromuscular impairment; pain; musculoskeletal impairment; perception or cognitive impairment; anxiety; decreased energy or fatigue.

Defining characteristics: Dyspnea; shortness of breath; tachypnea; fremitus; abnormal arterial blood gases; cyanosis; cough; nasal flaring; respiratory depth changes; purse-lip breathing; prolonged expiratory phase; increased anteroposterior diameter; use of accessory muscles; altered chest excursion; assumption of 3-point position.

RISK FOR INJURY

Definition: An individual is at risk of injury as a result of environmental conditions interacting with the individual's adaptive and defensive resources.

Related to the presence of risk factors:
Internal: biochemical: regulatory function (sensory dysfunction); abnormal blood profile; leukocytosis or leukopenia; altered clotting factors, thrombocytopenia; sickle cell-thalassemia; decreased hemoglobin; physical: (broken skin, altered mobility); developmental age; psychologic: (affective, orientation); [history of falls].

External: biologic: immunization level of the community; environmental pollutants; chemical: pollutants, poisons, drugs, pharmacologic agents (anesthetic agents, overdose CNS depressants), alcohol, caffeine, nicotine, preservatives, cosmetics and dyes, nutrients (vitamins, food types); physical: design, structure, and arrangement of community, building, or equipment; mode of transport or transportation; people/provider: nosocomial agents; staffing patterns; cognitive, affective, and psychomotor factors.

RISK FOR SUFFOCATION

Definitions: Accentuated risk of accidental suffocation (inadequate air available for inhalation).

Related to the presence of risk factors:
Internal: Reduced olfactory sensation; reduced motor abilities; lack of safety education and precautions (smoking in bed); cognitive or emotional difficulties; disease or injury process.

External (environmental): Pillow placed in an infant's crib; propped bottle placed in an infant's crib; warming car in closed garage; children playing with plastic bags or inserting small objects into their mouths or noses; discarded or unused refrigerators or freezers without removed doors; children left unattended in bathtubs or pools; household gas leaks; smoking in bed; use of fuel-burning heaters not vented to outside; low-strung clothesline; pacifier hung around infant's head; person who eats large mouthfuls of food [while talking or laughing].

RISK FOR POISONING

Definition: Accentuated risk of accidental exposure to or ingestion of drugs or dangerous products in doses sufficient to cause poisoning.

Related to the presence of risk factors:
Internal, the individual: Reduced vision; verbalization of occupational setting without adequate safeguards; lack of safety or drug education; lack of proper precaution, cognitive or emotional difficulties; insufficient finances.

External, the environmental: Large supplies of drugs in house; medicines stored in unlocked cabinets accessible to children or confused persons; dangerous products placed or stored within the reach of children or confused persons; availability of illicit drugs potentially contaminated by poisonous additives; flaking, peeling paint or plaster in presence of young children; chemical contamination of food and water; unprotected contact with heavy metals or chemicals; paints, lacquer, etc., in poorly ventilated areas or without effective protection; presence of poisonous vegetation; chemical contamination of food and water; presence of atmospheric pollutants.

RISK FOR TRAUMA

Definition: Accentuated risk of accidental tissue injury (wound, burn, fracture).

Related to the presence of risk factors:
Internal, the individual: Weakness; poor vision; balancing difficulties [unsteady gait, uncorrected visual problems]; reduced temperature or tactile sensation; reduced large- or small-muscle coordination; reduced hand-eye coordination; lack of safety education; lack of safely precautions; cognitive or emotional difficulties; history of previous trauma; insufficient finances to purchase safety equipment or effect repairs.

External, the environmental: Litter or liquid spills on floors or stairways (wet or highly waxed); snow or ice collected on stairs, walkways; unanchored rugs; bathtub without hand grip or antislip equipment; use of unsteady ladders or chairs; entering unlighted rooms; unsturdy or absent stair rails; unanchored electric wires; high beds; children playing without gates at the top of the stairs; obstructed passageways [hallways on hospital units]; unsafe window protection in homes with young children; inappropriate call-for-aid mechanisms [call light] for bed-resting client; pot handles facing toward front of stove; bathing in very hot water (unsupervised bathing of young children [and debilitated elderly]; potential igniting gas leaks; delayed lighting of gas burner or oven; experimenting with chemicals or gasoline; unscreened fires or heaters; wearing plastic apron or flowing clothes around open flame; children playing with matches, candles, cigarettes; inadequately stored combustible or corrosives, e.g., matches, oily rags, lye); highly flammable children's toys or clothing; overloaded fuse boxes; contact with rapidly moving machinery, industrial belts or pulleys; sliding on coarse bed linen; struggling within bed restraints [improperly applied restraints; failure to offer alternative measures to restraints]; faulty electrical plugs, frayed wires, or defective appliances; contact with acids or alkalis; playing with fireworks or gunpowder; contact with intense cold; overexposure to sun, sun lamps, radiotherapy; use of cracked dishware or glasses; knives stored uncovered; guns or ammunition stored unlocked; large icicles hanging from the roof; exposure to dangerous machinery; children playing with sharp-edged toys; high crime neighborhood and vulnerable clients; driving a mechanically unsafe vehicle; driving after partaking of alcoholic beverages or drugs; driving at excessive speeds; driving without necessary visual aids; children riding in front seat in car, [riding in car without infant safety seats]; smoking in bed or near oxygen; overloaded electrical outlets; grease waste collected on stoves; use of thin or worn potholders; misuse of necessary headgear for motor cyclists or young children carried on adult bicycles; [roller blading while pushing infant in stroller]; unsafe road or road-crossing conditions; play or work near vehicle pathways, e.g., driveways, laneways, railroad tracks; nonuse or misuse of seat restraints.

RISK FOR ASPIRATION

Definition: An individual is at risk for entry of gastrointestinal secretions, oropharyngeal secretions, or solids or fluids into tracheobronchial passages.

Related to the presence of risk factors: Reduced level of consciousness; depressed cough and gag reflexes; presence of tracheostomy or endotracheal tube; tube feedings; impaired swallowing; wired jaws; incomplete lower esophageal sphincter; gastrointestinal tubes; medication administration; situations hindering elevation of upper body; increased intragastric pressure; increased gastric residual; decreased gastrointestinal motility; delayed gastric emptying; impaired swallowing; facial/oral/neck surgery or trauma.

RISK FOR DISUSE SYNDROME

Definition: An individual is at risk for deterioration of body systems as the result of prescribed or unavoidable musculoskeletal inactivity. N. B: Complications from immobility can include pressure ulcers; constipation; stasis of pulmonary secretions; thrombosis; urinary tract infection or retention; decreased strength and endurance; orthostatic hypotension; decreased range of joint motion; disorientation; body image disturbance and powerlessness.

Related to the presence of risk factors: Paralysis; mechanical immobilization; severe pain; altered level of consciousness.

ALTERED PROTECTION

Definition: An individual experiences a decrease in the ability to guard the self from internal or external threats such as illness or injury.

Related factors: Extremes of age; inadequate nutrition; alcohol abuse; abnormal blood profiles e.g., leukopenia, thrombocytopenia; coagulation; anemia; immunosuppression; drug therapies (e.g., antineoplastic, corticosteroid, immune, anticoagulant, thrombolytic); treatments (e.g., surgery, radiation); and diseases such as cancer and immune disorders.

Defining characteristics: Deficit immunity; impaired healing; altered clotting; maladaptive stress response; neurosensory alteration; chilling; perspiring; fatigue.

IMPAIRED TISSUE INTEGRITY

Definition: An individual experiences damage to mucous membranes, corneal, integumentary, or subcutaneous tissue.

Related factors: Altered circulation; nutritional deficit or excess; fluid deficit or excess; knowledge deficit; impaired physical mobility; irritants, chemical, including body excretions, secretions, medications; thermal (e.g., temperature extremes); mechanical, pressure, shear, friction; radiation including therapeutic radiation.

Defining characteristics: Damaged or destroyed cornea, mucous membrane, integumentary, or subcutaneous tissue.

ALTERED ORAL MUCOUS MEMBRANE

Definitions: The state in which an individual experiences disruptions in the tissue layers of the oral cavity.

Related factors: Pathologic conditions: oral cavity, (e.g., radiation to the head or neck); dehydration; chemical trauma, (e.g., acidic foods, drugs, noxious agents, alcohol); mechanical trauma, e.g., ill fitting dentures, braces, endotracheal or nasogastric tubes; NPO for more than 24 hours; ineffective oral hygiene; mouth breathing; malnutrition; infection; medications; lack of or decreased salivation.

Defining characteristics: Oral pain or discomfort; coated tongue; xerostomia (dry mouth); stomatitis; oral lesions or ulcers; lack of or decreased salivation; leukoplakia; edema; hyperemia; desquamation; vesicles; oral plaque; carious teeth; halitosis; hemorrhagic gingivitis.

IMPAIRED SKIN INTEGRITY

Definitions: A state in which the individual's skin is adversely altered (e.g., shearing).

Related factors:

External, the environmental: hyper- or hypothermia; chemical substance; mechanical factors, e.g., shearing forces, pressure, restraint; radiation; physical immobilization.
Internal, the individual: Medications; obesity or emaciation; altered metabolic state; altered circulation; altered sensation; skeletal prominence; altered pigmentation; developmental factors; immunologic deficit; alterations in turgor, a change in elasticity.

Defining characteristics: Disruption of skin surface; destruction of skin layers; invasion of body structures.

RISK FOR IMPAIRED SKIN INTEGRITY

Definition: A state in which the individual's skin is at risk of being adversely altered.

Related to the presence of risk factors:

External environmental: hypo- or hyperthermia; chemical substances; mechanical factors (shearing forces, pressure, restraint); radiation; physical immobilization; excretions or secretions; humidity.
Internal, the individual: Medications; altered metabolic state; obesity or emaciation; altered sensation; skeletal prominence; psychogenic; immunologic; altered pigmentation; developmental factors; alterations in skin turgor, a change in elasticity.

DECREASED ADAPTIVE CAPACITY: INTRACRANIAL

Definition: A clinical state in which intracranial fluid dynamic mechanisms that normally compensate for increases in intracranial volumes are compromised, resulting in repeated disproportionate increase in intracranial pressure (ICP) in response to a variety of noxious and non-noxious stimuli.

Related factors: Brain injuries; sustained increase in ICP > 10–15 mm Hg; decreased cerebral perfusion pressure < 50–60 mm Hg; systemic hypotension with intracranial hypertension.

Defining characteristics: Repeated increase in ICP of greater than 10 mm Hg for more than 5 minutes following any of a variety of external stimuli.

ENERGY FIELD DISTURBANCE

Definition: A disruption of the flow of energy surrounding a person's being that results in a disharmony of the body, mind, or spirit.

Related factors: Inability to cope with life stressors; inability to manage behavior or anger.

Defining characteristics: Temperature change, warmth or coolness; visual changes, image or color; disruption of the field, vacant, hold, spike, bulge; movement, wave, spike, tingling, dense, flowing; sounds (tone or words).

IMPAIRED VERBAL COMMUNICATION

Definition: An individual experiences a decreased or absent ability to use or understand language in human interaction.

Related factors: Decrease in circulation to brain; physical barrier, a tracheostomy, intubation; anatomic defect, a cleft palate; psychologic barriers, psychosis, lack of stimuli; developmental or age-related; cultural difference [English as a second language].

Defining characteristics: Unable to speak dominant language; speaks or verbalizes with difficulty; does not or cannot speak; stuttering; slurring; difficulty forming words; difficulty expressing thoughts verbally; disorientation; inappropriate verbalization; dyspnea.

IMPAIRED SOCIAL INTERACTION

Definition: Insufficient or excessive quantity or ineffective quality of social exchange.

Related factors: Knowledge or skill deficit about ways to enhance mutuality; communication barriers; self-concept disturbance; absence of available significant others or peers; limited physical mobility; therapeutic isolation; environmental barriers; environmental barriers; altered thought processes.

Defining characteristics: Verbalized or observed discomfort in social situations; verbalized or observed inability to receive or communicate a satisfying sense of belonging, caring, interest, or shared history; observed use of unsuccessful social interaction behaviors; dysfunctional interactions with peers, family, or others.

SOCIAL ISOLATION

Definition: Aloneness experienced by the individual and perceived as imposed by others and as a negative or threatened state.

Related factors: Delay in accomplishing developmental tasks; immature interests; alterations in physical appearance; alterations in mental status; unaccepted social behavior; unaccepted social values; altered state of wellness; inadequate personal resources; inability to engage in satisfying personal relationships.

Defining characteristics: Absence of supportive significant other(s) such as family friends, group; sad dull affect; inappropriate or immature interest or activities for development age or stage; uncommunicative; withdrawn; no eye contact; preoccupation with own thoughts; repetitive meaningless actions; projects hostility in voice, behavior; seeks to be alone or exists in a subculture; evidence of physical or mental handicap or altered state of wellness; shows behavior unaccepted by dominant cultural group.

RISK FOR LONELINESS

Definition: A subjective state in which an individual is at risk of experiencing vague dysphoria [exaggerated feeling of depression and unrest without apparent cause].

Related factors: Affectional deprivation; physical isolation; cathectic deprivation [inability to concentrate psychic energy on some particular person, thing, or idea]; social isolation.

Defining characteristics: In research process: keeping to self; failure to interact with others.

ALTERED ROLE PERFORMANCE

Definition: Disruption in the way one perceives one's role performance.

Related factors: Situational or maturational crises; involuntary release from employment; death of spouse or significant other.

Defining characteristics: Change in self-perception; denial of role; change in others' perception of role; conflict in roles; changes in physical capacity to resume role; change in usual patterns of responsibility.

ALTERED PARENTING

Definition: The state in which a nurturing figure(s) experiences an inability to create an environment that promotes the optimum growth and development of another human being.

Related factors: Lack of available role model; ineffective role model; physical and psychosocial abuse of nurturing figure; lack of support between or from significant other(s); unmet social maturation needs of parenting figures; interruption in bonding process, e.g., maternal, paternal, other; unrealistic expectation of self, infant, partner; perceived threat to own survival, physical and emotional; interruption in bonding process; mental or physical illness; presences of stress, financial, legal, recent crisis, cultural move; lack of knowledge; limited cognitive functioning; lack of role identity; lack or inappropriate response of child to relationship; multiple pregnancies.

Defining characteristics: Abandonment; runaway; verbalization: cannot control child; incidence of physical and psychologic trauma; lack of parental attachment behaviors; inappropriate visual, tactile, auditory stimulation; negative identification of infant or child's characteristics; negative attachment of meanings to infant or child's characteristics; constant verbalization of disappointment in gender or physical characteristics of the infant or child; verbalization of resentment toward the infant or child; verbalization of role inadequacy; inattentive to infant's or child's needs; verbal disgust at body functions of infant or child; noncompliance with health appointments for self or infant or child; inappropriate caretaking behavior (toilet training, sleep and rest, feeding); inappropriate or inconsistent discipline practices; frequent accidents; history of child abuse or abandonment by primary caretaker; verbalizes desire to have child call him or herself by first name versus traditional cultural tendencies; child receives care from multiple caretakers without consideration for the needs of the infant or child; compulsively seeking role approval from others.

RISK FOR ALTERED PARENTING

Definition: The state in which a nurturing figure(s) is at risk to experience an inability to create an environment that promotes optimum growth and development of another human being.

Related to the presence of risk factors: Lack of available role model; lack of support between or from significant other; unmet social or emotional maturation needs of parenting figures; physical and psychosocial abuse of nurturing figure; interruption in bonding process (maternal, paternal, other); unrealistic expectation for self, infant, partner; perceived threat to own survival, physical and emotional; mental or physical illness; presence of stress (financial, legal, recent crisis, cultural move); lack of knowledge; limited cognitive functioning; lack of role identity; lack or inappropriate response of child to relationship; multiple pregnancies.

Defining characteristics: Lack of parental attachment behaviors; inappropriate visual, tactile, auditory stimulation; negative identification of infant or child's characteristics; negative attachment of meaning to infant or child's characteristics; constant verbalization of disappointment in gender or physical characteristics of the infant or child; verbalization of resentment toward the infant or child; verbalization of role inadequacy; inattentive to infant's or child's needs; verbal disgust at body functions of infant or child; noncompliance with health appointments for self or infant or child; inappropriate caretaking behaviors (toilet training, sleep and rest, feeding); inappropriate or inconsistent discipline practices; frequent accidents; frequent illness; growth and development lag in the child; positive history of child abuse or abandonment by primary caretaker; verbalized desire to have child call himself or herself by first name versus traditional cultural tendencies; child receives care from multiple caretakers without consideration for the needs of the infant or child; compulsively seeking role approval from others.

RISK FOR ALTERED PARENT/INFANT/CHILD ATTACHMENT

Definition: Disruption of the interactive process between parent or significant other and infant that fosters the development of a protective and nurturing reciprocal relationship.

Related to the presence of risk factors: Inability of parent to meet the personal needs; anxiety associated with the parent role; substance abuse; premature infant; ill infant or child who is unable to effectively initiate parental contact as a result of altered behavioral organization; separation; physical barriers; lack of privacy.

SEXUAL DYSFUNCTION

Definition: A change in sexual function that is viewed as unsatisfying, unrewarding, inadequate.

Related factors: Biopsychosocial alteration of sexuality; physical abuse; psychosocial abuse, harmful relationship; vulnerability; values conflict; lack of privacy; ineffectual or absent role models; lack of significant other; altered body structure or function, pregnancy, recent childbirth, drugs, surgery, anomalies, disease process, trauma, radiation; misinformation or lack of knowledge.

Defining characteristics: Verbalization of problem; alterations in achieving perceived sex role; actual or perceived limitation imposed by disease or therapy; conflicts involving values; alteration in achieving sexual satisfaction; inability to achieve desired satisfaction; seeking confirmation of desirability; alteration in relationship with significant other; change of interest in self and others.

ALTERED FAMILY PROCESSES

Definition: The state in which a family that normally functions effectively experiences a dysfunction.

Related factors: Situation transition or crisis; developmental transition or crisis.

Defining characteristics: Family system unable to meet physical and emotional needs of its members; family unable to adapt to traumatic experience constructively; family system unable to meet spiritual needs of its members; parents do not demonstrate respect for each other's views on child-rearing practices; inability to express or accept wide range of feelings; inability to express or accept feelings of members; family unable to meet security needs of its members; inability of the family members to relate to each other for mutual growth and maturation; family uninvolved in community activities; inability to accept or receive help appropriately; rigidity in function and roles; a family not demonstrating respect for individuality and autonomy of its members; family unable to adapt to change or deal with traumatic experience constructively; family failing to accomplish current or past developmental task; unhealthy family decision-making process; failure to send and receive clear message; inappropriate boundary maintenance; inappropriate or poorly communicated family rules, rituals, symbols; unexamined family myths; inappropriate level and direction of energy.

CAREGIVER ROLE STRAIN

Definition: A caregiver's felt difficulty in performing the family caregiver role.

Related factors:
Pathophysiologic/physiologic: Illness severity of the care receiver; addiction or codependency; premature birth or congenital defect; discharge of family member with significant home care needs; caregiver health impairment; unpredictable illness course or instability in the care receiver's health; caregiver is female; psychological or cognitive problems in care receiver.

Developmental: Caregiver is not developmentally ready for caregiver role (e.g., a young adult needing to provide for a middle-aged parent); developmental delay or retardation of the care receiver or caregiver.

Psychosocial: Psychologic or cognitive problems in care receiver; marginal family adaptation or dysfunction prior to the caregiving situation; marginal caregiver's coping patterns; past history of poor relationship between caregiver and care receiver; caregiver is spouse; care receiver exhibits deviant, bizarre behavior.

Situational: Presence of abuse or violence; presence of situational stressors that normally affect families (significant loss, disaster or crisis, poverty or economic vulnerability, major life events such as birth, hospitalization, leaving home, returning home, marriage, divorce, employment, retirement, death); duration of caregiving required (years); inadequate physical environment for providing care (housing, transportation, community services, equipment); family or caregiver isolation; lack of respite and recreation for caregiver; inexperience with caregiving; caregiver's competing role commitments; complexity or amount of caregiving tasks.

RISK FOR CAREGIVER ROLE STRAIN

Definition: A caregiver is vulnerable for felt difficulty in performing the family caregiver role.

Related to the presence of risk factors:
Pathophysiologic: Illness severity of the care receiver; addiction or codependency; premature birth or congenital defect; discharge of family member with significant home care needs; caregiver health impairment; unpredictable illness course or instability in the care receiver's health; caregiver is female; psychologic or cognitive problems in care receiver.

Developmental: Caregiver is not developmentally ready for caregiver role (young adult needs to provide care for middle-aged parent); developmental delay or retardation of the care receiver or caregiver.

Psychologic: Marginal family adaptation or dysfunction prior to the caregiving situation; marginal care-

giver's coping patters; past history of poor relationship between caregiver and care receiver; caregiver is spouse; care receiver exhibits deviant, bizarre behavior.

Situational: Presence of abuse or violence; presence of situational stressors that normally affect families, significant loss, disaster or crisis, poverty or economic vulnerability, major life events such as birth, hospitalization, leaving home, returning home, marriage, divorce, employment, retirement, death; duration of caregiving required [years]; inadequate physical environment for providing care, housing, transportation, community service, equipment; family or caregiver isolation; lack of respite and recreation for caregiver; inexperience with caregiving; caregiver's competing role commitment; complexity or amount of caregiving tasks.

ALTERED FAMILY PROCESS: ALCOHOLISM

Definition: The state in which the psychosocial, spiritual, and physiologic functions of the family unit are chronically disorganized, leading to conflict, denial of problems, resistance to change, ineffective problem solving, and a series of self-perpetuating crises.

Related factors: Abuse of alcohol; family history of alcoholism, resistance to treatment; inadequate coping skills, genetic predisposition; addictive personality; lack of problem-solving skills; biochemical influences.

Defining characteristics:
Major feelings: Decreased self-esteem and worthlessness; anger or suppressed rage; frustration; powerlessness; anxiety, tension, distress; insecurity; repressed emotions; responsibility for alcoholic's behavior; lingering resentment; shame and embarrassment; hurt; unhappiness; guilt; emotional isolation and loneliness; vulnerability; mistrust; hopelessness; rejection.

Roles and relationships: Deterioration in family relationships and disturbed family dynamics; ineffective spouse communication or marital problems; altered role function and disruption of family roles; inconsistent parenting or low perception of parental support; family denial; intimacy dysfunction; chronic family problems; closed communication systems.

Behaviors: Expression of anger inappropriately; difficulty with intimate relationships; loss of control of drinking; impaired communication; ineffective problem-solving skills; enabling to maintain drinking; inability to meet emotional needs of its members; manipulation; dependency; criticizing; alcohol abuse; broken promises; rationalization or denial of problems; refusal to get help or inability to accept and receive help appropriately; blaming; inadequate understanding or knowledge of alcoholism.

PARENTAL ROLE CONFLICT

Definition: The state in which a parent experiences role confusion and conflict in response to crisis.

Related factors: Separation from child resulting from chronic illness; intimidation with invasive or restrictive modalities (isolation, intubation); specialized care centers, policies; home care of a child with special needs (apnea monitoring, postural drainage, hyperalimentation); change in marital status; interruptions of family life due to home care regimen (treatments, caregivers, lack of respite).

Defining characteristics:
Major: Parent(s) expresses concern/feelings of inadequacy to provide for child's physical and emotional needs during hospitalization or in the home; demonstrated disruption in care taking routines; parent(s) expresses concerns about changes in parental role, family functioning, family communication, family health.
Minor: Expresses concern about perceived loss of control over decisions relating to the child; reluctant to participate in usual caretaking activities even with encouragement and support; verbalizes, demonstrates feelings of guilt, anger, fear, anxiety, or frustrations about effect of child's illness on family process.

ALTERED SEXUALITY PATTERNS

Definition: The state in which an individual expresses concern regarding his or her sexuality.

Related factors: Knowledge or skill deficit about alternative responses to health-related transitions, altered body function or structure, illness or medical problems; lack of privacy; impaired relationship with significant other; lack of significant other; ineffective or absent role models; altered body function; fear of acquiring a sexually transmitted disease; conflicts with sexual orientation or variant preferences; fear of pregnancy;

Defining characteristics: Reported difficulties, limitation, or changes in sexual behaviors or activities.

SPIRITUAL DISTRESS (DISTRESS OF THE HUMAN SPIRIT)

Definition: Disruption in the life principle that pervades a person's entire being and that integrates and transcends one's biologic and psychosocial nature.

Related factors: Separation from religious or cultural ties; challenged belief and value system (caused by moral or ethical implications of therapy, caused by intense suffering).

Defining characteristics: Expresses concern with meaning of life, death, and belief systems; anger toward God; questions meaning of suffering; verbalizes inner conflict about beliefs; verbalizes concern about relationship with deity; questions meaning of own existence; unable to participate in usual religious practices; seeks spiritual assistance; questions moral or ethical implications of therapeutic regimen; gallows humor [cynical humor]; displacement of anger toward religious representatives; description of nightmares or sleep disturbances; alteration in behavior or mood evidenced by anger, crying, withdrawal, preoccupation, anxiety, hostility, apathy.

POTENTIAL FOR ENHANCED SPIRITUAL WELL-BEING

Definition: Spiritual well-being is the process of an individual's developing or unfolding of mystery through harmonious interconnectedness that springs from inner strengths.

Defining characteristics: Inner strengths: a sense of awareness, self-consciousness, sacred source, unifying force, inner core, and transcendence; unfolding mystery: one's experience about life's purpose and meaning, mystery, uncertainty, and struggles; harmonious interconnectedness; relatedness, connectedness, harmony with self, others, higher power or God, and the environment.

INEFFECTIVE INDIVIDUAL COPING

Definition: Impairment of adaptive behaviors and problem-solving abilities of a person in meeting life's demands and roles.

Related factors: Situational crises; maturational crises; personal vulnerability.

Defining characteristics: Verbalization of inability to cope or inability to ask for help; inability to meet basic needs; inability to solve problems; high rate of accidents; alteration in society participation; destructive behavior toward self or others; inappropriate use of defense mechanisms; change in usual communication patterns; verbal manipulation; high illness rate; high rate of accidents.

IMPAIRED ADJUSTMENT

Definition: The state in which the individual is unable to modify his or her life-style or behavior in a manner consistent with a change in health status.

Related factors: Disability requiring change in lifestyle; inadequate support systems; impaired cognition; sensory overload; assault to self-esteem; altered locus of control; incomplete grieving.

Defining characteristics: Verbalization of nonacceptance of health status change; unsuccessful in goal setting; [expression of anger toward others].

DEFENSIVE COPING

Definition: The state in which an individual repeatedly projects falsely positive self-evaluation based on a self-protective pattern that defends against underlying perceived threats to positive self-regard.

Related factors: Anxiety; lack of problem-solving skills; perceived threat to self.

Defining characteristics: Denial of obvious problems or weaknesses; projection of blame or responsibility; rationalizes failures; grandiosity; hypersensitive to criticism.

INEFFECTIVE DENIAL

Definition: A conscious or unconscious attempt to disavow the knowledge or meaning of an event to reduce anxiety or fear to the detriment of health.

Related factors: Fear; substance abuse; perceived threat to self.

Defining characteristics: Delays seeking health care to the detriment of health; does not perceive personal relevance of symptoms or danger; uses home remedies to relieve symptoms.

INEFFECTIVE FAMILY COPING: DISABLING

Definition: Behavior of significant person, family member or other primary person that disables his or her own capacities and the client's capacities to effectively address tasks essential to either person's adaptation to the health challenge.

Related factors: Significant person with chronically unexpressed feelings of guilt, anxiety, hostility, despair; arbitrary handling of family's resistance to treatment; dissonant discrepancy of coping styles for dealing with adaptive task by the significant person and client or among significant people; highly ambivalent family relationships; arbitrary handling of family's resistance to treatment, which tends to solidify defensiveness, as it fails to deal adequately with underlying anxiety.

Defining characteristics: Neglectful care of client in regard to basic human needs or illness treatment; distortion of reality regarding the client's health problem, including extreme denial about its existence or severity; intolerance; rejection; abandonment; desertion; carrying on usual routines, disregarding needs; psychosomaticism; taking on illness signs of client; decisions and actions by family that are detrimental to economic or social well-being; agitation, depression, aggression, hostility; impaired restructuring of a meaningful life for self; impaired individualization; prolonged overconcern for client; neglectful relationships with other family members; client's development of helpless, inactive dependence; hostility.

INEFFECTIVE FAMILY COPING: COMPROMISED

Definition: A usually supportive primary person is providing insufficient, ineffective, or compromised support, comfort, assistance, or encouragement that may be needed by the client to manage or master adaptive tasks related to his or her health challenge.

Related factors: Progression of disease exhausts the supportive capacity of significant other; temporary family disorganization and role changes; incorrect information or understanding by a primary person; temporary preoccupation by a significant person who is trying to manage emotional conflicts and personal suffering and is unable to perceive or act effectively in regard to needs; temporary family disorganization and role changes; other situational or developmental crises or situations that significant person may be facing; little support provided by client, in turn, for primary person; prolonged disease or disability progression that exhausts supportive capacity of significant people.

Defining characteristics:
Subjective: Client expresses a concern about significant other's response to his or her health problem; significant person describes preoccupation with personal reaction (fear, anticipatory grief, guilt, anxiety to illness, disability, or to other situational or developmental crises); significant other confirms inadequate understanding of knowledge base that interferes with effective supportive behaviors; significant other withdraws into limited communication with client at the time of need.

FAMILY COPING: POTENTIAL FOR GROWTH

Definition: Effective managing of adaptive tasks by family member involved with the client's health challenge, who now is exhibiting desire and readiness for enhanced health and growth in regard to self and in relation to the client.

Related factor: Needs sufficiently gratified and adaptive tasks effectively addressed to enable goals of self-actualization to surface.

Defining characteristics: Family member attempting to describe growth impact of crisis on his or her own values, priorities, goals, or relationships; family member moving in direction of health-promoting and enriching life-style which supports and monitors maturational processes, audits and negotiates treatment programs, and generally chooses experiences that optimize wellness; individual expressing interest in making contact on a one-to-one basis or on a mutual-aid group basis with another person who has experienced a similar situation.

POTENTIAL FOR ENHANCED COMMUNITY COPING

Definition: A pattern of community activities for adaptation and problem solving that is satisfactory for meeting the demands or needs of the community but can be improved for management of current and future problems and stressors.

Related factors: Social supports available; resources available for problem solving; community has a sense of power to manage stressors.

Defining characteristics: Deficits in one or more characteristics that indicate effective coping; active planning by community for predicted stressors (hurricanes; earthquakes; fire-prone areas).

INEFFECTIVE COMMUNITY COPING

Definition: A pattern of community activities for adaptation and problem solving that is unsatisfactory for meeting the demands or needs of the community.

Related factors: Deficits in social support; inadequate resources for problem solving; powerlessness.

Defining characteristics: Community fails to meet its own expectations (unrealistic goal setting); deficits in community participation; excessive community conflicts; expressed difficulty in meeting demands for change; high illness rate [unsafe drinking water; air polluted by insecticides]; stressors perceived as excessive.

INEFFECTIVE MANAGEMENT OF THERAPEUTIC REGIMEN: INDIVIDUALS

Definition: A pattern of regulating and integrating into daily living a program for treatment of illness and the sequelae of illness that are unsatisfactory for meeting specific health goals.

Related factors: Complexity of health care system; complexity of therapeutic regimen; decisional conflicts; economic difficulties; excessive demands made on individual or family; family conflict; family patterns of health care; inadequate number and types of cues to action; knowledge deficits; mistrust of regimen or health care personnel; perceived seriousness; perceived susceptibility; perceived barriers; perceived benefits; powerlessness; social support deficits.

Defining characteristics: Choices of daily living ineffective for meeting the goals of a treatment or prevention program.

NONCOMPLIANCE (SPECIFY)

Definition: A person's informed decision not to adhere to a therapeutic recommendation.

Related factors: Patient value system: health beliefs, cultural influences, spiritual values; client-provider relationships.

Defining characteristics: Behavior indicative of failure to adhere (by direct observation or by statements of client or significant others); failure to keep appointments; [failure to follow therapeutic regimen]; objective tests (physiologic measures, detection of markers); evidence of development of complications; evidence of exacerbation of symptoms; failure to progress.

INEFFECTIVE MANAGEMENT OF THERAPEUTIC REGIMEN: FAMILIES

Definition: A pattern of regulating and integrating into family processes a program for treatment of illness and the sequelae of illness that is unsatisfactory for meeting specific health goals.

Related factors: Complexity of health care system; complexity of therapeutic regimen; decisional conflict; economic difficulties; excessive demand made on individual or family; family conflict.

Defining characteristics: Inappropriate family activities for meeting the goals of a treatment or prevention program.

INEFFECTIVE MANAGEMENT OF THERAPEUTIC REGIMEN: COMMUNITY

Definition: A pattern of regulating and integrating into community processes a program for treatment of illness and the sequelae of illness that is unsatisfactory for meeting health-related goals.

Defining characteristics: Deficits in persons and programs to be accountable for illness care of aggregates; deficits in advocates for aggregates; deficits in community activities for secondary and tertiary prevention; illness symptoms above the norm expected for the number and type of population; number of health care resources are insufficient for the incidence or prevalence of illness(es); unavailable health care resources for illness care; unexpected acceleration of illness(es).

EFFECTIVE MANAGEMENT OF THERAPEUTIC REGIMEN: INDIVIDUAL

Definition: A pattern of regulating and integrating into daily living a program for treatment of illness and its sequelae that is satisfactory for meeting specific health goals.

Defining characteristics: Appropriate choices of daily activities for meeting the goals of a treatment or prevention program; illness symptoms are within a normal range of expectation; verbalized desire to manage the treatment of illness and prevention of sequelae; verbalized intent to reduce risk factors for progression of illness and sequelae.

DECISIONAL CONFLICT (SPECIFY)

Definition: The state of uncertainty about course of action to be taken when choice among competing actions involves risk, loss, or challenge to personal life values.

Related factors: Unclear personal values; perceived threat to value system; support system deficit; lack of relevant information; multiple or divergent sources of information.

Defining characteristics: Verbalized uncertainty about choices; verbalization of undesired consequences of alternative actions being considered; vacillation between alternative choices; delayed decision making.

HEALTH SEEKING BEHAVIORS (SPECIFY)

Definition: A state in which an individual in stable health is actively seeking ways to alter personal health habits, or the environment in order to move toward a higher level of health.

Related factors: Desire to achieve an optimal state of wellness and well-being.

Defining characteristics: Expressed or observed desire to seek a higher level of wellness; unfamiliarity with wellness resources in the community.

IMPAIRED PHYSICAL MOBILITY

Definition: A state in which the individual experiences a limitation of ability for independent physical movement.

Related factors: Intolerance of activity; decreased strength and endurance; pain or discomfort; perceptual or cognitive impairment; neuromuscular impairment; musculoskeletal impairment; depression or severe anxiety.

Defining characteristics: Inability to purposefully move within the physical environment; limited range of motion; decreased muscle strength; imposed restrictions of movement (chemical or physical restraints); impaired coordination.

Functional Level Classification
0 = Completely independent
1 = Required use of equipment or device
2 = Requires help from another person, for assistance, supervision, or teaching
3 = Requires help from another person and equipment device
4 = Dependent, does not participate in activity

RISK FOR PERIPHERAL NEUROVASCULAR DYSFUNCTION

Definition: A state in which an individual is at risk of experiencing a disruption in circulation, sensation, or motion of an extremity.

Related to the presence of risk factors: Fractures; mechanical compression (tourniquet, cast, brace, dressing or restraints; orthopedic surgery; trauma; immobilization; burns; vascular obstruction).

RISK FOR PERIOPERATIVE POSITIONING INJURY

Definition: A state in which the client is at risk for injury as a result of the environmental conditions found in the perioperative setting.

Related to the presence of risk factors:
Disorientation; immobilization, muscle weakness; sensory or perceptual disturbances resulting from anesthesia; obesity; emaciation; edema.

ACTIVITY INTOLERANCE

Definition: A state in which an individual has insufficient physiologic or psychologic energy to endure or complete required or desired daily activities.

Related factors: Bed rest; immobility; generalized weakness; sedentary life-style; imbalance between oxygen supply and demand.

Defining characteristics: Verbal report of fatigue or weakness; abnormal heart rate or blood pressure response to activity; exertional discomfort or dyspnea; electrocardiographic changes reflecting arrhythmias or ischemia.

FATIGUE

Definition: An overwhelming sustained sense of exhaustion and decreased capacity for physical and mental work.

Related factors: Decreased or increased metabolic energy production; overwhelming psychologic or emotional demands; increased energy requirements to perform activity of daily living; altered body chemistry (medications, drug withdrawal, chemotherapy); excess social or role demands; states of discomfort.

Defining characteristics: Verbalization of an unremitting and overwhelming lack of energy; inability to maintain usual routines.

RISK FOR ACTIVITY INTOLERANCE

Definition: Individual is at risk of experiencing insufficient physiologic or psychologic energy to endure or complete required or desired daily activities.

Related to the presence of risk factors: History of previous intolerance; deconditioned status; presence of circulatory or respiratory problems; inexperience with the activity.

SLEEP PATTERN DISTURBANCE

Definition: Disruption of sleep time causes discomfort or interferes with desired life-style.

Related factors:
Internal: Sensory alterations resulting from illness, psychologic stress
External: Environmental changes; social cues.

Defining characteristics: Verbal complaints of difficulty falling asleep; awakening earlier or later than desired; interrupted sleep; verbal complaints of not feeling well-rested; lethargy; ptosis; expressionless face; dark circles under eyes; frequent yawning; changes in posture; thick speech with mispronunciation and incorrect words.

DIVERSIONAL ACTIVITY DEFICIT

Definition: An individual experiences a decreased stimulation from or interest or engagement in recreational or leisure activities.

Related factors: Environmental lack of diversional activity (long-term hospitalization, frequent lengthy treatments).

Defining characteristics: Client's statements regarding boredom; usual hobbies cannot be undertaken in hospital.

IMPAIRED HOME MAINTENANCE MANAGEMENT

Definition: Inability to independently maintain a safe growth-promoting immediate environment.

Related factors: Individual or family member disease or injury; insufficient family organization or planning; insufficient finances; unfamiliarity with community resources; impaired cognitive or emotional functioning; lack of knowledge; lack of role modeling; inadequate support systems.

Defining characteristics:
Subjective: Household members express difficulty in maintaining their home in a comfortable fashion; household members request assistance with home maintenance; household members describe outstanding debts or financial crises.
Objective: Unwashed or unavailable cooking equipment, clothes or linen; accumulation of dirt, food wastes, or hygienic wastes; offensive odors; inappropriate household temperature; overtaxed family members (exhausted, anxious); lack of necessary equipment

or aids; presence of vermin or rodents; repeated hygienic disorders, infestations, or infections.

ALTERED HEALTH MAINTENANCE

Definition: Inability to identify, manage, or seek out help to maintain health.

Related factors: Lack of or significant alteration in communication skills, written, verbal, or gestural; lack of ability to make deliberate and thoughtful judgments; perceptual or cognitive impairment, complete or partial lack of gross or fine motor skills; ineffective individual or family coping; lack of material resources; dysfunctional grieving; unachieved developmental tasks; disabling spiritual distress.

Defining characteristics: Demonstrated lack of knowledge regarding basic health practices; demonstrated lack of adaptive behaviors to internal or external environmental changes; reported or observed lack of equipment and finances; reported or observed impairment of personal support systems; reported or observed inability to take responsibility for meeting basic health practices in any or all functional pattern areas; history of lack of health-seeking behavior.

FEEDING SELF-CARE DEFICIT

Definition: An individual experiences an impaired ability to perform or complete feeding activities for self.

Related factors: Intolerance to activity, decreased strength and endurance; pain, perceptual, or cognitive impairment; neuromuscular impairment; musculoskeletal impairment; depression; severe anxiety.

Defining characteristics: Inability to bring food from a receptacle to the mouth.

IMPAIRED SWALLOWING

Definition: Decreased ability to voluntarily pass fluids or solids from the mouth to the stomach.

Related factors: Neuromuscular impairment (decreased or absent gag reflex; decreased strength or excursion of muscles involved in mastication; perceptual impairment; facial paralysis); mechanical obstruction (edema; tracheostomy tube; tumor); fatigue; limited awareness; reddened, irritated oropharyngeal cavity.

Defining characteristics: Observed evidence of difficulty in swallowing (stasis of food in oral cavity; coughing or choking).

INEFFECTIVE BREAST-FEEDING

Definition: The state in which a mother, infant, or child experience dissatisfaction or difficulty with the breast-feeding process.

Related factors: Prematurity; infant anomaly; maternal breast anomaly; maternal anxiety or ambivalence; previous breast surgery; previous history of breast-feeding failure; infant receiving supplemental feedings with artificial nipple; poor infant sucking reflex; nonsupportive partner or family; knowledge deficit; interruption in breast-feeding.

Defining characteristics: Unsatisfactory breast-feeding process; actual or perceived inadequate milk supply; infant inability to attach onto maternal breast correctly; insufficient emptying of each breast per feeding; persistence of sore nipples beyond the first week of breast-feeding.

INTERRUPTED BREAST-FEEDING

Definition: A break in the continuity of the breast-feeding process as a result of inability or inadvisability to put baby to breast for feeding.

Related factors: Maternal or infant illness; prematurity; maternal employment; contraindication to breast-feeding (drugs, true breast-milk jaundice); need to abruptly wean infant.

Defining characteristics: Infant does not receive nourishment at the breast for some or all of feedings; separation of mother and infant.

EFFECTIVE BREAST-FEEDING

Definition: The state in which a mother-infant dyad or family exhibits adequate proficiency and satisfaction with breast-feeding process.

Related factors: Basic breast-feeding knowledge; normal breast structure; normal infant oral structure; infant gestational age greater than 34 weeks; support sources; maternal confidence.

Defining characteristics: Mother able to position infant at breast to promote a successful latch-on response; infant is content after feeding; regular and sustained suckling and swallowing at the breast; appropriate infant weight patterns for age; effective mother-infant communication patterns (infant cues, maternal interpretation and response).

INEFFECTIVE INFANT FEEDING PATTERN

Definition: A state in which an infant demonstrates an impaired ability to suck or coordinate the suck-swallow response.

Related factors: Prematurity; neurologic impairment or delay; oral hypersensitivity; prolonged NPO; anatomic abnormality.

Defining characteristics: Inability to initiate or sustain an effective suck; inability to coordinate sucking, swallowing, and breathing.

BATHING/HYGIENE SELF-CARE DEFICIT

Definition: A state in which the individual experiences an impaired ability to perform or complete bathing or hygiene activities for self.

Related factors: Intolerance of activity, decreased strength and endurance; pain, discomfort; perceptual or cognitive impairment; neuromuscular impairment; musculoskeletal impairment; depression; severe anxiety.

Defining characteristics: Inability to wash body or body parts; inability to obtain or get to water source; inability to regulate temperature or flow.

DRESSING/GROOMING SELF-CARE DEFICIT

Definition: An impaired ability to perform or complete dressing and grooming activities for oneself.

Related factors: Intolerance of activity; decreased strength and endurance; pain, discomfort; perceptual or cognitive impairment; neuromuscular impairment; musculoskeletal impairment; depression; severe anxiety.

Defining characteristics: Impaired ability to put on or take off necessary items of clothing; impaired ability to obtain or replace articles of clothing; impaired ability to fasten clothing; inability to maintain appearance at a satisfactory level.

TOILETING SELF-CARE DEFICIT

Definition: An impaired ability to perform or complete toileting activities for oneself.

Related factors: Impaired transfer ability; impaired mobility status; intolerance of activity; decreased strength and endurance; pain, discomfort; perceptual or cogni-

tive impairment; neuromuscular impairment; musculoskeletal impairment; depression; severe anxiety.

Defining characteristics: Unable to get to toilet or commode; unable to sit on or rise from toilet or commode; unable to manipulate clothing for toileting; unable to carry out proper toilet hygiene; unable to flush toilet or commode.

ALTERED GROWTH AND DEVELOPMENT

Definition: An individual demonstrates deviations in norms from his or her age group.

Related factors: Inadequate caretaking; indifference; inconsistent responsiveness; multiple caretakers; separation from significant others; environmental and stimulation deficiencies; effects of physical disability; prescribed dependence.

Defining characteristics: Delay of difficulty in performing skills (motor, social, or expressive) typical of age group; altered physical growth; inability to perform self-care or activities for age.

RELOCATION STRESS SYNDROME

Definition: Physiologic or psychosocial disturbances as a result of transfer from one environment to another.

Related factors: Past, concurrent, and recent losses; losses involved with decision to move; feeling of powerlessness; lack of adequate support system; little or no preparation for the impending move; moderate to high degree of environmental change; history and types of previous transfers; impaired psychosocial health status; decreased physical health status.

Defining characteristics:
Major: Change in environment or location; anxiety; apprehension; increased confusion (elderly population: depression; loneliness).
Minor: Verbalization of unwillingness to relocate; sleep disturbance; change in eating habits; dependency; gastrointestinal disturbances; increased verbalization of needs; insecurity; lack of trust; restlessness; sad affect; unfavorable comparison of post/pre-transfer staff; verbalization of being concerned or upset about transfer; vigilance; weight change; withdrawal.

RISK FOR DISORGANIZED INFANT BEHAVIOR

Definition: Risk for alteration in integration and modulation of the physiologic and behavioral systems of functioning (autonomic, motor, state, organizational, self-regulatory, and attentional-interactional systems).

Risk factors: Pain; oral or motor problems; environmental overstimulation; lack of containment and boundaries; prematurity; invasive or painful procedures.

DISORGANIZED INFANT BEHAVIOR

Definition: Risk for alteration in integration and modulation of the physiologic and behavioral systems of functioning (autonomic, motor, state, organizational, self-regulatory, and attentional-interactional systems).

Related to the presence of risk factors: Pain; oral or motor problems; feeding intolerance; environmental overstimulation; lack of containment or boundaries; prematurity; invasive or painful procedures.

Defining characteristics: Change from baseline physiologic measures; tremors, startles, twitches; hyperextension of arms and legs; diffuse sleep; deficient self-regulatory behavior; deficient response to visual or auditory stimuli.

POTENTIAL FOR ENHANCED ORGANIZED INFANT BEHAVIOR

Definition: A pattern of modulation of the physiologic and behavioral systems of functioning of an infant (autonomic, motor, state, organizational, self-regulatory) and attentional-interactional systems, that is satisfactory but that can be improved, resulting in higher levels of integration in response to environmental stimuli.

Related factors: Prematurity; pain.

Defining Characteristics: Stable physiologic measures; definite sleep-wake states; use of some self-regulatory behaviors; response to visual and auditory stimuli.

BODY IMAGE DISTURBANCE

Definition: Disruption in the way one perceives one's body image.

Related factors: Biophysical; cognitive or perceptual; psychosocial; cultural or spiritual.

Defining characteristics: Evidence required for this diagnosis is (a) verbal response to actual or perceived change in structure or function (fear of rejection or reaction by others); and (b) nonverbal response to actual or perceived change in structure or function.

Subjective: Preoccupation with loss; personalization of the part by name; depersonalization of the part by impersonal pronouns; refusal to verify actual change.

Objective: Missing body part; actual change in structure or function; not looking at part; not touching body part; inability to estimate spatial relationship of body to environment; change in social involvement [refusal to attend social functions formerly enjoyed].

SELF-ESTEEM DISTURBANCE

Definition: Negative self-evaluation or feelings about self or self-capabilities, which may be directly or indirectly expressed.

Related factors: History of physical, sexual, or verbal abuse: disintegrated thought processes; unmet dependency needs; retarded ego development; dysfunctional family support system.

Defining characteristics: Self-negating verbalization; expressions of shame or guilt; evaluates self as unable to deal with events; rationalizes away or rejects positive feedback and exaggerates negative feedback about self; hesitant to try new things or situations; denial of problems obvious to others; projection of blame or responsibility for problems; rationalizing personal failures; hypersensitive to criticism; grandiosity.

CHRONIC LOW SELF-ESTEEM

Definition: Long standing negative self-evaluation or feelings about self or self capabilities.

Related factors: History of physical, sexual, or verbal abuse: disintegrated thought processes; unmet dependency needs; retarded ego development; dysfunctional family support system.

Defining characteristics:
Major: Long standing or chronic manifestation of self-negating verbalization; expressions of shame or guilt; evaluates self as unable to deal with events; rationalizes away or rejects positive feedback and exaggerates negative feedback about self; hesitant to try new things or situations.
Minor: Frequent lack of success in work or other life events; overly conforming, dependent on others' opinions; lack of eye contact; nonassertive or passive; indecisive; excessively seeks reassurance.

SITUATIONAL LOW SELF-ESTEEM

Definition: Negative self-evaluation or feelings about self that develop in response to a loss or change in an individual who previously had a positive self-evaluation.

Related factors: Loss of employment; change in family support system; change in cognitive processes; change in physical abilities.

Defining characteristics: Episodic occurrence of negative self-appraisal in response to life events in a person with a previous positive self-evaluation; verbalization of negative feelings about the self (hopelessness, uselessness); [perceived inability to make further contributions to family and community].

PERSONAL IDENTITY DISTURBANCE

Definition: Inability to distinguish between self and nonself. Diagnosis requires further research. The following are the author's comments:

Related factors: Disintegration of ego boundaries; disintegration of thought processes; unmet dependency needs; retarded ego development.

Defining characteristics: Extreme mood changes; inability to define self-boundaries; inability to give direction to life or set goals; presence of more than one personality within the individual.

SENSORY/PERCEPTUAL ALTERATIONS (specify: visual, auditory, kinesthetic, gustatory, tactile, olfactory)

Definition: An individual experiences a change in the amount or patterning of oncoming stimuli accompanied by a diminished, exaggerated, distorted, or impaired response to such stimuli.

Related factors: Altered environmental stimuli (excessive or insufficient); altered sensory reception, transmission, or integration; chemical alteration from electrolyte imbalance or medications; psychologic stress.

Defining characteristics: Disoriented to time, place, or person; altered abstraction; altered conceptualization; change in problem-solving abilities; reported or measured change in sensory acuity; change in behavior patterns; altered communication patterns; anxiety; apathy; change in usual response to stimuli; indication of body-image alteration; restlessness; irritability.

UNILATERAL NEGLECT

Definition: An individual is perceptually unaware or inattentive to one side of the body.

Related factors: Effects of disturbed perceptual abilities (hemianopia, or one-sided blindness; neurologic illness or trauma).

Defining characteristics: Consistent inattention to stimuli on an affected side.

HOPELESSNESS

Definition: An individual sees limited or no alternatives or personal choices available and is unable to mobilize energy on own behalf.

Related factors: Prolonged activity restriction creating isolation; failing or deteriorating physiologic condition; long-term stress; abandonment; lost belief in transcendent values or God.

Defining characteristics: Passivity, decreased verbalization; decreased affect; verbal cues of despondence ("I can't.").

POWERLESSNESS

Definition: Perception that one's own action will not significantly affect an outcome; a perceived lack of control over a current situation or immediate happening.

Related factors: Health care environment; interpersonal interaction; illness-related regimen; life-style of helplessness.

Defining characteristics: Verbal expressions of having no control or influence over situation; verbal expressions of having no control or influence over outcome; verbal expressions of having no control over self-care; depression over physical deterioration that occurs despite client compliance with regimens; apathy.

KNOWLEDGE DEFICIT

Definition: Absence or deficiency of cognitive information related to specific topic.

Related factors: Lack of exposure; lack of recall; information misinterpretation; cognitive limitation; lack of interest in learning; unfamiliarity with information resources.

Defining characteristics: Verbalization of the problem; inaccurate follow-through of instruction; inaccurate performance of test; inappropriate or exaggerated behavior (hysterical, hostile, agitated, apathetic).

IMPAIRED ENVIRONMENTAL INTERPRETATION SYNDROME

Definition: Consistent lack of orientation to person, place, time, or circumstances (situations) over more than 3 to 6 months necessitating a protective environment.

Related factors: Dementia (Alzheimer's disease, multi-infarct dementia, Pick's disease, AIDS dementia); Parkinson's disease; Huntington's disease; depression; alcoholism.

Defining characteristics: Consistent disorientation in known and unknown environments; chronic confusional states.

ACUTE CONFUSION

Definition: The abrupt onset of a cluster of global, transient changes and disturbances in attention, cognition, psychomotor activity, level of consciousness, or sleep-wake cycle.

Related factors: Over 60 years of age; dementia; alcohol abuse; drug abuse; delirium.

Defining characteristics: Fluctuation in cognition; fluctuation in sleep-wake cycle; fluctuation in level of consciousness; fluctuation in psychomotor activity; increased agitation or restlessness; misperceptions; lack of motivation to initiate or follow through with goal-directed or purposeful behavior.

CHRONIC CONFUSION

Definition: An irreversible, long-standing, or progressive deterioration of intellect and personality characterized by decreased ability to interpret environmental stimuli, decreased capacity for intellectual thought processes, and manifested by disturbances of memory, orientation, and behavior.

Related factors: Alzheimer's disease; Korsakoff's psychosis; multi-infarct dementia; cerebral vascular accident; head injury.

Defining characteristics:
Major: Clinical evidence of organic impairment; altered interpretation of or response to stimuli; progressive or long-standing cognitive impairment.
Minor: No change in level of consciousness; impaired socialization; impaired memory (short term, long term); altered personality.

ALTERED THOUGHT PROCESSES

Definition: An individual experiences a disruption in cognitive operations and activities. Diagnosis requires further research to identify related to factors. The following are the author's comments:

Related factors: Cognitive distortions; developmental lag; sensory overload; substance abuse.

Defining characteristics: Inappropriate non–reality-based thinking; inaccurate interpretation of environment; cognitive dissonance; distractibility; memory deficit; egocentricity; hyper- or hypovigilance.

IMPAIRED MEMORY

Definition: The state in which an individual experiences the inability to remember or recall bits of information or behavioral skills. Impaired memory may be attributed to pathophysiologic or situational causes that are either temporary or permanent.

Related factors: Acute or chronic hypoxia; anemia; decreased cardiac output; fluid and electrolyte imbalance; neurologic disturbances; excessive environmental disturbances.

Defining characteristics: Observed or reported experiences of forgetting; inability to determine if a behavior was performed; inability to learn or retain new skills or information; inability to perform a previously learned skill; inability to recall factual information; inability to recall recent or past events.

PAIN

Definition: An individual experiences and reports the presence of severe discomfort or an uncomfortable sensation.

Related factors: Injury agents (biologic, chemical, physical, psychologic).

Defining characteristics:
Subjective: Communication (verbal or coded) of pain descriptors.
Objective: Guarding behavior, protective; self-focusing; narrowed focus (altered time perception, withdrawal from social contact, impaired thought process); distraction behavior (moaning, crying, pacing, seeking out other people, restlessness); facial mask of pain (eyes lackluster, beaten look, fixed or scattered movement, grimace); alteration in muscle tone (may span from listless to rigid); autonomic responses not seen in

chronic stable pain (diaphoresis, blood pressure and pulse change, pupillary dilation, increased or decreased respiratory rate).

CHRONIC PAIN

Definition: The individual experiences pain that continues for more than 6 months duration.

Related factors: Chronic physical or psychosocial disability.

Defining characteristics: Verbal report or observed evidence of pain experienced for more than 6 months; fear of another injury; physical and social withdrawal.

DYSFUNCTIONAL GRIEVING

Definition: Extended, unsuccessful use of intellectual and emotional responses by which individuals attempt to work through the process of modifying self-concept based upon the perception of loss.

Related factors: Actual or perceived object loss (*object lost* is used in the broadest sense); objects may include people, possessions, job, status, home, ideals, parts and processes of the body.

Defining characteristics: Verbal expressions of distress at loss; denial of loss; expression of guilt; expression of unresolved issues; anger; crying; difficulty in expressing loss; expression of feeling sad all the time; alterations in eating habits, dream patterns, activity level, libido; idealization of lost object; reliving of past experiences; interference with life functioning; developmental regression; labile affect; alterations in concentration or pursuits of tasks.

ANTICIPATORY GRIEVING

Definition: Intellectual and emotional responses and behaviors by which individuals work through the process of modifying self-concept based on the perception of potential loss.

Related factors: Expectation of a loss.

Defining characteristics: Potential loss of significant object; expression of distress at potential loss; denial of potential loss; expressions of guilt, anger, sorrow, choked feelings; changes in libido; changes in eating habits; alterations in sleep patterns, activity level, communication.

RISK FOR VIOLENCE; SELF-DIRECTED OR DIRECTED AT OTHERS

Definition: An individual experiences behaviors that can be physically harmful either to the self or others.

Related to presence of risk factors: Antisocial character; battered women; catatonic excitement; child abuse; manic excitement; organic brain syndrome; panic state; rage reactions; suicidal behavior; temporal lobe epilepsy; toxic reactions to medication.

Defining characteristics: Body language (clenched fists, facial muscles tautness indicating effort to control, rigid posture); hostile threatening verbalizations (boasting of abuse to others); increased motor activity (pacing, excitement, irritability, agitation); overt and aggressive acts (goal-directed destruction of objects in environment); possession of destructive means (gun, knife, weapon); rage; self-destructive behavior; active aggressive suicidal acts; suspicion of others; paranoid ideation; delusions; hallucinations; substance abuse or withdrawal.

RISK FOR SELF-MUTILATION

Definition: A state in which an individual is at risk to perform an act upon the self to injure, not kill, which produces tissue damage and tension relief.

Related to the presence of risk factors:
Groups at risk: Clients with borderline personality disorder, especially women 16–25 years of age; clients in psychotic state, frequently men in young adulthood; emotionally disturbed or battered children; mentally retarded and autistic children; clients with a history of self-injury; history of physical, emotional, or sexual abuse.

Defining characteristics: Inability to cope with increased psychologic or physiologic tension in a healthy manner; feelings of depression, rejection, self-hatred, separation anxiety, guilt, and depersonalization; fluctuating emotions; command hallucination; need for sensory stimuli; parental emotional deprivation; dysfunctional family.

POST-TRAUMA RESPONSE

Definition: An individual experiencing a sustained painful response to an overwhelming traumatic event(s).

Related factors: Disasters, wars, epidemics, rape, assault, torture, catastrophic illness or accident.

Defining characteristics: Reexperience of the traumatic event, which may be identified in cognitive, affective, or sensory motor activities (flashbacks, intrusive thoughts, repetitive nightmares, excessive verbalization of the traumatic event, verbalization of survival guilt).

RAPE-TRAUMA SYNDROME

Definition: Forced violent sexual penetration against the victim's will and consent. The trauma syndrome that develops from this attack or attempted attack includes an acute phase of disorganization of the victim's life-style and a long-term process of reorganization of life-style.

Related factors: Sexual abuse.

Defining characteristics:
Acute phase: Emotional reactions (anger, embarrassment, fear of physical violence and death, humiliation, revenge, self-blame); multiple physical symptoms (gastrointestinal irritability, genitourinary discomfort, muscle tension, sleep pattern disturbance).

Long-term reactions: Changes in life-style (change in residence, repetitive nightmares and phobias, seeking family support, seeking social network support).

RAPE-TRAUMA SYNDROME: COMPOUND REACTION

Definition: See rape-trauma syndrome.

Related factors: Sexual abuse.

Defining characteristics: See rape-trauma syndrome. Reactivated symptoms of previous conditions such as physical illness, psychiatric illness, reliance on alcohol or drugs.

RAPE-TRAUMA SYNDROME: SILENT REACTION

Definition: See rape-trauma syndrome.

Related factors: Sexual abuse.

Defining characteristics: Abrupt changes in relationships with men; increase in nightmares; increased anxiety during interview (blocking of associations, long periods of silence, minor stuttering, physical distress); pronounced changes in sexual behavior; no verbalization of the occurrence of rape; sudden onset of phobic reactions.

ANXIETY

Definition: A vague uneasy feeling whose source is often nonspecific or unknown to the individual.

Related factors: Unknown conflict about essential values or goals of life; threat to self-concept; threat of death; threat to or change in health status; threat to or change in role functioning; threat to or change in environment; threat to or change in interaction patterns; situational or maturational crises; interpersonal transmission or contagion; unmet needs.

Defining characteristics:
Subjective: Increased tension; apprehension; painful and persistent increased helplessness; uncertainty; fearful; scared; regretful; overexcited; rattled; distressed; jittery; feelings of inadequacy; shakiness; fear of unspecific consequences; expressed concerns about change in life events; worried; anxious.

Objective: Sympathetic stimulation such as cardiovascular excitation, superficial vasoconstriction, pupil dilation; restlessness; insomnia; poor eye contact; trembling; facial muscles taut; voice quivering.

FEAR

Definition: Feeling of dread related to an identifiable source that the person validates.

Related factors: Lack of support system; lack of knowledge; language barrier; sensory impairment.

Defining characteristics: Ability to identify object of fear.

Appendix C
Nursing Diagnoses Grouped by Gordon's 11 Functional Health Patterns

HEALTH PERCEPTION-HEALTH MANAGEMENT PATTERN
- Altered health maintenance
- Altered protection
- Health-seeking behaviors (specify)
- Ineffective management of therapeutic regimen (individual)
- Effective management of therapeutic regimen (individual)
- Ineffective management of therapeutic regimen (family)
- Ineffective management of therapeutic regimen (community)
- Noncompliance (specify)
- Risk for infection
- Risk for injury
- Risk for poisoning
- Risk for suffocation
- Risk for trauma
- Risk for perioperative positioning injury

NUTRITIONAL-METABOLIC PATTERN
- Altered nutrition: potential for more than body requirements.
- Altered nutrition: more than body requirements
- Altered nutrition: less than body requirements
- Effective breast-feeding
- Interrupted breast-feeding
- Ineffective breast-feeding
- Ineffective infant eating pattern
- Impaired swallowing
- Risk for aspiration
- Altered oral mucous membranes
- Risk for fluid volume deficit
- Fluid volume deficit
- Fluid volume excess
- Risk for impaired skin integrity
- Impaired skin integrity
- Impaired tissue integrity
- Risk for altered body temperature
- Ineffective thermoregulation
- Hyperthermia
- Hypothermia

ELIMINATION PATTERN
- Constipation
- Perceived constipation
- Colonic constipation
- Diarrhea
- Bowel incontinence
- Altered urinary elimination pattern
- Stress incontinence
- Reflex incontinence
- Urge incontinence
- Functional incontinence
- Total incontinence
- Urinary retention

ACTIVITY-EXERCISE PATTERN
- Risk for activity intolerance
- Activity intolerance (specify level)
- Fatigue
- Impaired physical mobility (specify level)
- Risk for disuse syndrome
- Total self-care deficit (specify level)
- Bathing/hygiene self-care deficit (specify level)
- Dressing/grooming self-care deficit (specify level)
- Feeding self-care deficit (specify level)
- Toileting self-care deficit (specify level)
- Diversional activity deficit
- Impaired home maintenance management (mild, moderate, severe, high-risk, chronic)
- Dysfunctional ventilatory weaning response (DVWR)
- Ineffective airway clearance
- Ineffective breathing pattern
- Impaired gas exchange
- Decreased cardiac output
- Altered tissue perfusion (specify: renal, cerebral, cardiopulmonary, gastrointestinal, peripheral)
- Dysreflexia
- Altered growth and development
- Risk for peripheral neurovascular dysfunction

SLEEP-REST PATTERN
- Sleep pattern disturbance

COGNITIVE-PERCEPTUAL PATTERN
- Pain
- Chronic pain
- Sensory/perceptual alterations: input deficit or sensory deprivation
- Sensory/perceptual alterations: input excess or sensory overload
- Unilateral neglect
- Knowledge deficit (specify)
- Impaired thought processes
- Decisional conflict (specify)
- Decreased adaptive capacity: intracranial
- Risk for disorganized infant behavior
- Disorganized infant behavior
- Potential for enhanced organized infant behavior
- Impaired environmental interpretation syndrome
- Acute confusion

- Chronic confusion
- Impaired memory

SELF-PERCEPTION AND SELF-CONCEPT PATTERN
- Fear
- Anxiety
- Hopelessness
- Powerlessness (severe, low, moderate)
- Body image disturbance
- Self-esteem disturbance
- Chronic low self-esteem
- Situational low self-esteem
- Personal identity disturbance
- Risk for self-mutilation
- Energy field disturbance

ROLE-RELATIONSHIP PATTERN
- Anticipatory grieving
- Dysfunctional grieving
- Disturbance in role performance
- Social isolation
- Risk for loneliness
- Impaired social interaction
- Altered family processes
- Altered family process: alcoholism
- Altered parenting
- Risk for altered parenting
- Parental role conflict
- Impaired verbal communication
- Risk for violence
- Relocation stress syndrome
- Risk for altered parent/infant/child attachment
- Caregiver role strain

SEXUALITY-REPRODUCTIVE PATTERN
- Sexual dysfunction
- Altered sexuality patterns
- Rape-trauma syndrome
- Rape-trauma syndrome: compound reaction
- Rape-trauma syndrome: silent reaction

COPING AND STRESS-TOLERANCE PATTERN
- Ineffective individual coping
- Impaired adjustment
- Defensive coping
- Ineffective denial
- Post-trauma response
- Ineffective family coping: disabling

- Ineffective family coping: compromised
- Family coping: potential for growth
- Potential for enhanced community coping
- Ineffective community coping

VALUE-BELIEF PATTERN

- Spiritual distress (distress of the human spirit)
- Potential for enhanced spiritual well-being

Appendix D
Nursing Diagnoses Grouped by a Modified Body Systems Approach

Suggested grouping of nursing diagnoses using a modified body systems approach.

MUSCULOSKELETAL, Rest, Sleep
- Activity intolerance
- High risk for activity intolerance
- Diversional activity deficit
- Sleep pattern disturbance
- Dysreflexia
- Fatigue
- Risk for disuse syndrome
- Altered protection
- Impaired physical mobility
- Risk for suffocation
- Risk for injury
- Risk for trauma
- Risk for aspiration
- Risk for perioperative positioning injury

CARDIOVASCULAR
- Decreased cardiac output
- Altered tissue perfusion

GASTROINTESTINAL, GENITOURINARY
- Constipation
- Perceived constipation
- Colonic constipation
- Diarrhea
- Bowel incontinence
- Altered urinary elimination pattern
- Stress incontinence
- Reflex incontinence

- Urge incontinence
- Functional incontinence
- Total incontinence
- Urinary retention
- Risk for aspiration

INTEGUMENTARY, FOOD, FLUID
- Fluid volume excess
- Fluid volume deficit
- Risk for fluid volume deficit
- Altered nutrition: more than body requirements
- Altered nutrition: less than body requirements
- Altered nutrition: potential for more than body requirements
- Altered oral mucous membrane
- Impaired swallowing
- Effective breast-feeding
- Ineffective breast-feeding
- Feeding self-care deficit
- Impaired tissue integrity
- Impaired skin integrity
- Risk for impaired skin integrity
- Interrupted breast-feeding
- Ineffective infant feeding pattern

NEUROLOGIC, EYE, EAR, PAIN
- Impaired verbal communication
- Unilateral neglect
- Sensory/perceptual alterations: input deficit or sensory deprivation
- Sensory/perceptual alterations: input excess or sensory overload
- Impaired thought processes

- Pain
- Chronic pain
- Risk for trauma
- Risk for injury
- Risk for aspiration
- Decreased adaptive capacity: intracranial
- Impaired environmental interpretation syndrome
- Acute confusion
- Chronic confusion
- Impaired memory

RESPIRATORY
- Impaired gas exchange
- Ineffective airway clearance
- Ineffective breathing pattern

REPRODUCTIVE
- Sexual dysfunction
- Altered sexuality patterns

ENDOCRINE
- Risk for altered body temperature
- Hypothermia
- Hyperthermia
- Ineffective thermoregulation

PSYCHIATRIC, PSYCHOLOGIC
- Ineffective individual coping
- Impaired adjustment
- Defensive coping
- Ineffective denial
- Decisional conflict (specify)
- Anxiety
- Fear
- Dysfunctional grieving
- Anticipatory grieving
- Hopelessness
- Powerlessness
- Post-trauma response
- Rape-trauma syndrome
- Rape-trauma syndrome: compound reaction
- Rape-trauma syndrome: silent reaction
- Body image disturbance
- Self-esteem disturbance
- Chronic low self-esteem
- Situational low self-esteem
- Personal identity disturbance

- Spiritual distress (distress of the human spirit)
- Energy field disturbance
- Relocation stress syndrome
- Risk for disorganized infant behavior
- Disorganized infant behavior
- Risk for self-mutilation

CURRENT HEALTH PROMOTION PRACTICES
- Bathing/hygiene self deficit
- Dressing/grooming self-care deficit
- Toileting self-care deficit
- Altered growth and development
- Knowledge deficit (specify)
- Noncompliance (specify)
- Risk for infection
- Altered health maintenance
- Impaired home maintenance management
- Health-seeking behaviors (specify)
- Risk for injury
- Risk for suffocation
- Risk for poisoning
- Risk for trauma
- Risk for aspiration
- Ineffective management of therapeutic regimen: families
- Ineffective management of therapeutic regimen: community
- Effective management of therapeutic regime: individual

HOME SITUATION AND RELATIONSHIP WITH OTHERS
- Ineffective family coping: disabling
- Ineffective family coping: compromised
- Family coping: potential for growth
- Impaired social interaction
- Social isolation
- Altered role performance
- Altered parenting
- Potential altered parenting
- Altered family processes
- Parental role conflict
- Risk for violence: self-directed or directed at others
- Risk for altered parent/infant/child attachment
- Caregiver role strain
- Risk for caregiver role strain
- Altered family process: alcoholism
- Potential for enhanced spiritual well-being
- Potential for enhanced community coping
- Ineffective community coping

Appendix E
List of Measurable Verbs and Criteria

Measurable verbs reflect the client's and nurse's actions that are seen, heard, felt, or smelled. The list is a guide and is not conclusive. Measurable verbs are written in the outcomes, nursing interventions, and nurses' notes.

SEE	HEAR	FEEL	SMELL
ambulate	auscultate	feel	emit
assess	communicate	finger	inhale
cough	consult	handle	smell
deep breath	delegate	palpate	sniff
demonstrate	describe	stroke	whiff
document	discuss	touch	
drink	explain		
eat	identify		
examine	list		
exercise	listen		
expectorate	participate		
implement	percuss		
measure	refer		
monitor	respond		
observe	reinforce		
perform	reiterate		
record	report		
redemonstrate	review		
turn	teach		
wash	state		
	verbalize		

Nonspecific verbs are not measurable. This list is a guide and is not conclusive. Avoid using nonspecific verbs in the outcomes, nursing interventions, and nurses' notes.

accept	ensure	have	poor
allow	facilitate	know	put
alter	fair	inadequate	restrict
do	feel	learn	try
employ	frequent	let	use
enable	get	limit	
encourage	good	permit	

Criteria serve as gauges of the client's progress in achieving the outcomes. The list is not inclusive.

accurately	willingly
independently	with assistance
realistically	walks to bathroom (10 feet)
within identified physio-	and back unassisted
logical parameters	while awake
(e.g., BP < 130/80)	without falling
safely	5 min every hour
unassisted	

Appendix F
List of Normal Values: Blood, Urine, Stool

This list of normal values contains information for use in answering the exercises in case studies #1 and #2. The list is not inclusive. Refer to other resources for additional information.

CHEMISTRIES

Source of specimen: serum, plasma, whole blood

TEST	NORMAL VALUE
Albumin	3.5–5.0 g/dL
Blood urea nitrogen	See Urea nitrogen
Calcium (Ca^{++})	9–11 mg/dL
Carbon dioxide (CO_2 content)	20–30 mEq/L
Chloride (Cl^-)	95–105 mEq/L
Cholesterol	150–250 mg/dL varies with age
Creatinine	0.5–1.5 mg/dL
Glucose, fasting	70–120 mg/dL
Potassium (K^+)	3.5–5.5 mEq/L
Sodium (Na^+)	135–145 mEq/L
Transaminase: Serum glutamic-oxaloacetic (SGOT); now called serum asparate amino-transferase (AST)	15–45 U/L
Urea nitrogen (BUN)	10–30 mg/dL

HEMATOLOGY

Red blood cells (RBC)	Male: 4.5–6.0 million/µL (mm³) Female: 4.0–5.0 million/µL (mm³)
Erythrocyte sedimentation rate (ERS)	Male: < 15 mm/h Female: < 20 mm/h
Hematocrit (Hct)	Male: 40–54% Female: 38–47%
Hemoglobin (Hbg)	Male: 13.5–18.0 g/dL Female: 12.0–16.0 g/dL
Prothrombin time (PT)	12–15 seconds (s) Values depend on reagent used
White blood cell count (WBC)	5000–10,000/µL (mm³)

SEROLOGY-IMMUNOLOGY

Human immunosuppressive virus (HIV)	Negative
Rheumatoid arthritis factor (RA factor)	Negative or titer < 1:20
VDRL	Nonreactive

TOXICOLOGY OF COMMON DRUGS

Salicylate level	Negative Therapeutic level: 15–30 mg/dL

CHARACTERISTICS OF NORMAL FECES

Color	Brown
Consistency	Formed; moist
Odor	Aromatic; affected by ingested food

CHARACTERISTICS
OF NORMAL FECES (CONT.)

Frequency	Varies from 1–3 movements per day to once every 3 days
Shape	Cylindrical
Amount	100–400 g/d (varies with diet)
Fat content	< 6 g/24 h
Mucus	Negative
Blood	Negative
Pus	Negative
Parasites	Negative

CHARACTERISTICS
OF NORMAL URINE

Amount in 24 hours	1200–1500 mL
Color	Straw, amber
Consistency	Clear liquid
Odor	Faint aromatic
Sterility	No microorganisms present
pH	4.5–8
Specific gravity	1.003–1.030
Glucose	Negative
Ketone bodies (acetone)	Negative
Blood	Negative

DIAGNOSTIC STUDIES

X-Ray findings	
Chest	Negative
Bones	Joint spaces within normal limits; negative for bony erosion, cartilage loss, and cysts
Electrocardiogram (ECG)	Normal sinus rhythm
Mammogram	Negative for masses
Skin test	Negative for allergens

Appendix G
Vital Signs, Height, and Weight for Adults

AVERAGE VITAL SIGNS BY AGE

AGE	TEMP	PULSE PER MIN	RESPIRATIONS PER MIN	BP
18 and over	37°C (98.6°F)	70–75	15–20	120/80
65 and over	36°C (96.8°F)	70–75	15–20	140/90

HEIGHT-WEIGHT TABLES,* METROPOLITAN 1983

Men					Women				
Height		Small Frame	Medium Frame	Large Frame	Height		Small Frame	Medium Frame	Large Frame
Feet	Inches				Feet	Inches			
5	2	128–134	131–141	138–150	4	10	102–111	109–121	118–131
5	3	130–136	133–143	140–153	4	11	103–113	111–123	120–134
5	4	132–138	135–145	142–156	5	0	104–115	113–126	122–137
5	5	134–140	137–148	144–160	5	1	106–118	115–129	125–140
5	6	136–142	139–151	146–164	5	2	108–121	118–132	128–143
5	7	138–145	142–154	149–168	5	3	111–124	121–135	131–147
5	8	140–148	145–157	152–172	5	4	114–127	124–138	134–151
5	9	142–151	148–160	155–176	5	5	117–130	127–141	137–155
5	10	144–154	151–163	158–180	5	6	120–133	130–144	140–159
5	11	146–157	154–166	161–184	5	7	123–136	133–147	143–163
6	0	149–160	157–170	164–188	5	8	126–139	136–150	146–167
6	1	152–164	160–174	168–192	5	9	129–142	139–153	149–170
6	2	155–168	164–178	172–197	5	10	132–145	142–156	152–173
6	3	158–172	167–182	176–202	5	11	135–148	145–159	155–176
6	6	162–176	171–187	181–207	6	0	138–151	148–162	158–179

Weight according to frame (ages 25–59) for men wearing indoor clothing weighing 5 lbs., shoes with one-inch heels; for women, indoor clothing weighing 3 lbs., shoes with one-inch heels.

* Reprinted with permission from the Metropolitan Life Insurance Company, New York.

Appendix H
Normal Values and Standards: Fluid Balance in an Adult

This information will assist students in answering the workbook's exercises. The lists of normal standards and values is not inclusive. Refer to other textbooks for further information.

NORMAL FLUID BALANCE IN THE ADULT

Intake	mL
Fluids	1200
Solid food	1000
Water from oxidation	300
Total	2500

Output	mL
Insensible loss (skin and lungs)	900
In feces	100
Urine	1500
Total	2500

COMMONLY USED FLUID CONTAINERS AND THEIR VOLUMES

Water glass	200 mL
Juice glass	120 mL
Cup	180 mL
Soup bowl	
Adult	180 mL
Child	100 mL
Teapot	240 mL
Creamer	
Large	90 mL
Small	30 mL
Water pitcher	1000 mL
Jello, custard dish	100 mL
Ice cream dish	120 mL
Paper cup	
Large	200 mL
Small	120 mL

Appendix I
Medications

The following list of medications is intended to assist the student in answering the exercises in case study #1 and case study #2.

Drug: Metaproterenol sulfate (**Alupent**)
Action: Beta-adrenergic stimulator, smooth-muscle relaxant, bronchodilator.
Uses: Asthma, bronchospasm.
Route: Oral, adults 20 mg every 6 to 8 hours. Inhalation, adults two or three inhalations, usually not repeated more often than every 3 or 4 hours. Total daily dosage should not exceed twelve inhalations. Each metered dose from inhaler delivers 0.65 mg metaproterenol.
Side effects: Nervousness, tachycardia, tremor, nausea.

Drug: Diphenhydramine hydrochloride (**Benadryl**)
Action: Antihistamine.
Uses: Relief of allergic conditions; in anaphylaxis as adjunct to epinephrine.
Route: Oral, intramuscular, intravenous.
Dosage: 25–50 mg three to four times a day. Maximum daily dosage 400 mg.
Side effects: Drowsiness, dizziness, headache, palpitation, dry mouth.

Drug: Docusate sodium (**Colace**)
Action: Stool softener, reduces surface tension.
Uses: Constipation; and clients who should avoid straining during defecation.
Route: Oral.
Dosage: Oral: Adults 50–200 mg/d, adjusted according to individual response.
Side effects: Bitter taste.

Drug: Cortisone acetate
Action: Anti-inflammatory.
Uses: Corticosteroid, glucocorticoid, mineralocorticoid.
Route: Oral, intramuscular.
Dosage: Individualized. Adult: initial oral dose 25–300 mg/qd. Dose reduced by periodic decrements of 10 to 25 mg/qd to lowest effective amount.
Side effects: Sodium and water retention. Increased blood pressure due to retention fluids. Hypokalemia. Suppressed immune response. Increased susceptibility to infection.

Drug: Acetylsalicylic acid (**Ecotrin**)
Action: Analgesic, anti-inflammatory, antipyretic.
Uses: Enteric coated aspirin; long-term aspirin therapy; antiarthritic; antiplatelet.
Route: Oral.
Dosage: Maximum daily dosage 4000 mg divided dosages (e.g., two 325 mg tablets every 4 hours).
Side effects: Gastric irritation and bleeding; increased bleeding time; ecchymosis; ringing in ears.

Drug: Ergotamine tartrate (**Ergomar, Ergostat, Ergotamine**)
Action: Vasoconstrictor; alpha-adrenoreceptor antagonist.
Uses: Antimigraine.
Route: Sublingual.
Dosage: At start of migraine, sublingual tablet 1–2 mg followed by another 1–2 mg at 30- to 60-minute intervals until at-

tack has abated. Dosage should not exceed 6 mg/24 h.

Side effects: Nausea, vomiting, diarrhea, weakness of legs, numbness and tingling fingers and toes.

Drug: Methotrexate (**Mexate, Folex**)
Action: Antineoplastic, antimetabolic, folic acid antagonist.
Uses: Principally used in combination regimens to maintain induced remissions in neoplastic diseases.
Route: Oral, intramuscular, intravenous, intra-arterial, intrathecal.
Dosage: Dosage individualized. Orally, 2.5 mg–5.0 mg/d. Treatment course of 5 days.
Side effects: Oral lesions. Gastrointestinal irritation. Hepatic toxicity. Blood dyscrasias. Photosensitivity.

Drug: Psyllium hydrophilic mucilloid (**Metamucil**)
Action: Bulk forming.
Uses: Constipation.
Route: Oral.
Dosage: 1–2 rounded teaspoonfuls one to three times daily; mix in 8 ounces (240 mL) water.
Side effects: Nausea, vomiting, diarrhea with excessive use.

Drug: Nafcillin (**Unipen**)
Action: Antibiotic.
Uses: Treatment of infections caused by penicillinase-producing *Staphylococcus aureus.*
Route: Oral, intramuscular, intravenous.
Dosage: Adults: 250 mg to 1 g orally every 4 to 6 hours; 500 mg intramuscularly every 4 to 6 hours; 500 mg to 1 g intravenously every 4 hours.
Side effects: Nausea, vomiting diarrhea, urticaria, pruritus.

Drug: Temazepam (**Restoril**)
Action: Hypnotic.
Uses: Relieve insomnia.
Route: Oral.
Dosage: Adult 15 to 30 mg at bedtime.
Side effects: Anorexia, diarrhea, drowsiness, lethargy.

Drug: Acetaminophen 300 mg with codeine phosphate 30 mg per tablet (**Tylenol #3**)
Action: Nonsalicylate analgesic and antipyretic. Combines the analgesic effects of a centrally acting analgesic, codeine, with a peripherally acting analgesic, acetaminophen.
Uses: Relief of mild to moderately severe pain.
Route: Oral.
Dosage: Adults, one or two tablets every 4 hours or as required (prn).
Side effects: Light-headedness, dizziness, sedation, shortness of breath, nausea and vomiting, hepatotoxicity.

Drug: Diclofenac sodium (**Voltaren**)
Action: Nonsteroid, anti-inflammatory analgesic and antipyretic.
Uses: Acute and chronic treatment of rheumatoid arthritis.
Route: Oral.
Dosage: Enteric-coated tablets. Rheumatoid arthritis, 150–200 mg/qd in divided doses, 50 mg three times a day (tid) or 75 mg twice a day (bid).
Side effects: Gastrointestinal toxicity such as bleeding, ulceration, and perforation can occur without warning.

Appendix J
Nonpharmacologic Pain Management: Relaxation Exercises

The purpose of relaxation exercises is to reduce high levels of stress and chronic and acute pain. The exercises are applicable to the clients in case studies #1 and #2. Relaxation techniques enable clients to exert control over their body's responses to tension and anxiety. This strategy has been used by women to relax during labor.

Exercise 1. Slow, rhythmic breathing for relaxation. Teach the client:

1. Breathe in slowly and deeply.
2. As you breathe out slowly, feel yourself beginning to relax; feel the tension leaving your body.
3. Now breathe in and out slowly and regularly, at whatever rate is comfortable for you. You may wish to try abdominal breathing.
4. To help you focus on your breathing slowly and rhythmically, breathe in as you say silently "in goes peace;" breathe out as you say silently, "out goes stress [or] pain."
5. May repeat steps for up to 20 minutes.

6. End with a slow deep breath. As you breathe out, say to yourself, "I feel alert and relaxed."

Exercise 2. Active listening to recorded music combined with imagery—a distraction exercise.

1. Obtain a tape recorder or compact disc (CD) player for the client, or check if it is permissible to play soothing music on the overhead speaker between 2000–2100, prior to sleep.
2. Tastes in music vary. Allow the client the option to make their own selections.
3. Clients may change music several times before finding a selection that they perceive assists them to relax.
4. Clients may adjust the music to a comfortable volume.
5. While the client is listening to the music, suggest that he or she imagine, with eyes closed, a seashore scene, walking in the woods, or a past experience that left him or her with a feeling of contentment.

Appendix K
ANA Standards of Clinical Nursing Practice (1991)

STANDARDS OF CARE

I. Assessment
   The Nurse collects client health data.
II. Diagnosis
   The Nurse analyzes the assessment data in determining diagnoses.
III. Outcome Identification
   The Nurse identifies expected outcomes individualized to the client.
IV. Planning
   The Nurse develops a plan of care that prescribes interventions to attain expected outcomes.
V. Implementation
   The Nurse implements the interventions identified in the plan of care.
VI. Evaluation
   The Nurse evaluates the client's progress toward attainment of outcomes.

STANDARDS OF PROFESSIONAL PERFORMANCE

I. Quality of Care
   The Nurse systematically evaluates the quality and effectiveness of nursing practice.

II. Performance Appraisal
   The Nurse evaluates his or her own nursing practice in relation to professional practice standards and relevant statutes and regulations.
III. Education
   The Nurse acquires and maintains current knowledge in nursing practice.
IV. Collegiality
   The Nurse contributes to the professional development of peers, colleagues, and others.
V. Ethics
   The Nurse's decisions and actions on behalf of clients are determined in an ethical manner.
VI. Collaboration
   The Nurse collaborates with the client, significant others, and health care providers in providing client care.
VII. Research
   The Nurse uses research findings in practice.
VIII. Resource Utilization
   The Nurse considers factors related to safety, effectiveness, and cost in planning and delivering client care.

* From *Standards of Clinical Nursing Practice.* Washington, DC: American Nurses Association; 1991. Used with permission.

Appendix L
Interdisciplinary Plan of Care

CLIENT WITH DIABETES MELLITUS

Client's name __Charles Durham__   DOB __7/5/30__   Medical Record Number __61580__   Date plan initiated __9/5/97__

Medical diagnosis(es) __Diabetes mellitus__   Nursing Diagnosis(es) __Ineffective management of therapeutic regimen__

Inpatient ____YES __X__ NO   Average length of stay _____   Case Manager __Samuel Cohn, RN__

Outpatient __X__ YES ____NO   Last clinic visit __6/16/97__   Primary physician/team __Julia George, MD__

Educational level __Completed high school__   Durable Power of Attorney __X__ YES ____NO   Living Will __X__ YES, location __medical record__ ____NO   Code status __X__ Full ____DNR

Client reviewed and agreed with plan __X__ YES ____NO ____NA, explain _____   Client's signature __Charles Durham__   Date __9/5/97__

Family reviewed and agreed with plan __X__ YES ____NO ____NA, explain _____   Family signature __Martha Durham (wife)__   Date __9/5/97__

CONTINUUM OF CARE

SITE: __X__ HOME ____NURSING HOME ____HOSPICE ____BOARD/CARE ____ADULT DAY CARE ____Homeless ____OTHER, SPECIFY _____

CAREGIVER: __X__ SPOUSE __X__ CHILDREN, SPECIFY __Son visits 1x/wk__ ____HEALTH AIDE ____NONE ____OTHER, SPECIFY _____

PROBLEM/ DIAGNOSIS/ DEFICIT	INTERDISCIPLINARY INTERVENTIONS	OUTCOMES	DATE MET	RESPONSIBLE DISCIPLINE	RESPONSIBLE PERSON/TITLE	DATE PLAN REVIEWED BY TEAM
Ineffective management of therapeutic regimen related to lack of understanding of diabetes mellitus.	Teach client and family disease process of diabetes mellitus.	Client and family will verbalize the disease process accurately.	9/8/97	Physician Nursing	Julia George, MD Samuel Cohn, RN	9/5/97 9/12/97
	Schedule monthly clinic visits with MD, and telephone calls to client weekly by RN.	Client adheres to regimen at home.	Ongoing	Physician Nursing	Julia George, MD Samuel Cohn, RN	10/7/97
Noncompliance with prescribed diabetic regimen.	Teach foot care.	No foot lesions throughout duration of care.	Ongoing	Nursing Physician	Samuel Cohn, RN Julia George, MD	
	Teach rationale for ADA diet.	Laboratory values WNL. Records daily food intake in diet diary.	9/12/97 9/12/97	Dietitian Physician	Lei Chen, RDT Julia George, MD	
Knowledge deficit: medications.	Teach insulin injection, types, dosage, times of administration, site rotation, storage of insulin.	Demonstrates injection technique accurately; verbalized knowledge of action of insulin.	9/5/97	Nursing	Samuel Cohn, RN	
Knowledge deficit: blood and urine testing.	Teach reason, technique for testing urine and blood, timing, recording results, required supplies.	Monitors glucose levels in blood and urine accurately.	9/12/97	Nursing Laboratory	Samuel Cohn, RN James Stuart, Laboratory technician	

Nursing diagnosis	Intervention	Goal/Outcome	Date	Discipline	Signature
Knowledge deficit: complications.	Teach clinical manifestations of hyperglycemia and hypoglycemia; the cause and treatment.	Client and wife verbalize accurately signs and symptoms hyperglycemia and hypoglycemia and treatment.	9/12/97	Nursing Physician	Samuel Cohn, RN Julia George, MD
Alteration in health maintenance related to lack of exercise.	Plan individualized exercise program with client. Review steps to prevent hyper- and hypoglycemia.	Participation in planned exercise program to improve muscle tone and endurance.	10/5/97	Physical therapy Occupational therapy Nursing	Beatrice Zane, PT Beatrice Zane, OT Samuel Cohn, RN
Safety measures.	Refer client to medical supplies for Medic-Alert identification band and diabetic alert card for wallet.	Verbalizes plan of action for self in event of illness. Verbalizes signs and symptoms requiring immediate interventions.	9/12/97	Nursing	Samuel Cohn, RN
High risk for infection.	Teach signs and symptoms of infection. Teach preventive measures.	Verbalizes signs and symptoms of infection and need for physician. Schedule annual dental, and physician visits.	9/12/97	Nursing Physician	Samuel Cohn, RN Julia George, MD

Date _____

Initial _____

Signature and Title _____

Appendix M

M-1: Vaginal Delivery
Critical Pathway: Infant

M-2: Vaginal Delivery
Critical Pathway: Mother

Appendix N

N-1: Cesarean Delivery
Critical Pathway: Infant

N-2: Cesarean Delivery
Critical Pathway: Mother

M-1
Vaginal Delivery
Critical Pathway: Infant

Date of Birth:_____   **Time of Birth:**_____

	0-6 Hours	7-12 Hours	13-18 Hours
Laboratory/ Diagnostic Tests	☐ Coombs ☐ Maternal Hep B status		
Treatments/ Procedures	☐ Stabilization ☐ Baby ID ☐ Vital signs as per patient standard ☐ Weight = _____ gm ☐ Bath	☐ Circumcision permit ☐ Hep B permit	
Medications/IVs	☐ Triple dye to cord ☐ Vitamin K ☐ Erythromycin ointment to eyes	☐ HBIG if mother Hep B positive or status unknown ☐ Hep B vaccine	
Consultations			
Activity	☐ Radiant warmer until stable temp	Open crib	Open crib
Nutrition	☐ Breastfeeding/or Glucose H2O	Breastfeeding per policy / care plan or formula at least q 4hrs	
Assessments	☐ Apgar at 1 and 5 minutes ☐ Gestational age ☐ Nursing assessment for VS, feeding, voiding, bonding	☐ I + O ☐ Nursing assessment for VS, feeding, voiding, bonding	☐ I + O ☐ Assess circumcision site
Education/ Discharge Planning	☐ See mother pathway		
Home Care			
Variances *Order*	☐	☐	☐
Reason			
Order	☐	☐	☐
Reason			

RN Signature: _____   _____   _____

_____   _____   _____

_____   _____   _____

Target discharge status =   Feeding well _____
Maintaining temperature _____
Voiding & stooling adequately _____
Bonding _____

Target LOS= 24-48 Hours

	19-24 Hours	Within 2 Hours of Discharge	Home 24-48 Hrs. Post Discharge
Laboratory/ Diagnostic Tests	◄········ PKU and bilirubin at age 24 hours ········► Coombs results Maternal RPR status at delivery		PKU, if initial PKU done before 24 hrs Bilirubin if > 5 at age 24 hours or if baby jaundiced by home health nurse; report results to by pediatrician
Treatments/ Procedures	Circumcision care if circumcision done		
Medications/IVs			
Consultations			
Activity	Open crib	Open crib	
Nutrition	Breast–feeding/or formula at least q 4hrs	Breast–feeding/or formula	
Assessments	Physician assessment of body systems Nursing assessment for VS, feeding, voiding, stooling, bonding		HHC nurse assessment of physical environment and baby, including VS, feeding, voiding, stooling, bonding, jaundice
Education/ Discharge Planning		Instructions to parents	
Home Care			
Variances *Order*			
Reason			
Order			
Reason			

Confirmed by pediatrician:

_____   _____
Signature   Date

Source: Thomas Jefferson University Hospital; Women and Children Care Program; Philadelphia

M-2
Vaginal Delivery
Critical Pathway: Mother

Date of Birth: _____

	Prenatal Record to L&D by 36 weeks	Labor, Delivery, Recovery	0-12 Hours
Laboratory/ Diagnostic Tests	☐ H + H ☐ Type + Screen ☐ Rubella ☐ RPR ☐ HBSAG	☐ CBC per order ☐ MS BOS per order ☐ RPR	☐ H+H or CBC if ordered ☐ Determine Rhogam and Rubella status

Treatments/ Assessments		☐ Receive medical record from MD's
		    office by 36 weeks
		☐ Assessment, vital signs and EFM
		    per patient care standard
			☐ Post partum assessment per
			    patient care standard
			☐ Peri care
			☐ Hygiene + comfort measures
			☐ Anesthesia follow-up if indicated

Medications/IVs	☐ Prenatal vitamins	☐ Analgesia/Anesthesia per order ☐ Pitocin per order	☐ IV discontinued ☐ Analgesics as needed for pain
Consultations	☐ Social Work per guidelines		☐ Lactation consult if breastfeeding ☐ Social Work PRN ☐ Pediatrician visit with mother ···▶
Activity		☐ OOB unless contraindicated	☐ OOB with assistance ☐ Shower ☐ Voiding without difficulty ☐ Rest
Nutrition	☐ Appropriate weight gain	☐ Clear liquids per order ☐ Ice	☐ Regular diet

Education/ Discharge Planning	☐ Childbirth preparation classes
	☐ Parentcraft classes
	☐ Breast–feeding class if BF
	☐ Orient to discharge program tour
	☐ Contraceptive planning
	☐ Select pediatrician
	☐ *Preparing for Your Baby's Birth*
	    at Jefferson
	☐ "Baby Talk" video
		☐ Comfort measures and
		    relaxation techniques
		☐ Orient to EFM
		☐ 2nd stage pushing
		☐ Initial breast–feeding instruction
		    if breast–feeding
		☐ Breast–feeding
			☐ Handwashing
			☐ Orient to baby's crib
			☐ Infant positioning, feeding,
			    changing

Home Care	☐ Referral to home care		
Variances *Order* *Reason* *Order* *Reason* *Order* *Reason*			

RN Signature: _____   _____   _____

_____   _____   _____

_____   _____   _____

Target discharge status = Minimal vaginal bleeding
Demonstrates parenting skills
Minimal physical discomfort

Target Post Delivery LOS = 24-48 Hours

Time of Birth:_____

	13-24 Hours	Within 2 hrs. of Discharge	Home
Laboratory/ Diagnostic Tests	☐ Rhogam if Rh negative and baby Rh positive ☐ RPR results ☐ Rubella if not immune		
Treatments/ Assessments	☐ Assess parenting skills ☐ Post partum assessment per patient care standard ☐ Peri care ☐ Hygiene + comfort measures ☐ Anesthesia follow-up if indicated		☐ Follow-up phone call at 3-5 days post discharge by maternity nurse to assess ☐ Assessment by HHC nurse
Medications/IVs	☐ Stool softener as ordered ☐ Analgesics as needed for pain		
Consultations	☐ problem (per BF Care Plan and Supplementation Policy/Procedure) ----------------------------------▶		☐ Lactation consult if breast-feeding problem ☐ Social work consult if needed
Activity	☐ OOB with assistance ☐ Voiding without difficulty ☐ Rest	☐ Escort mother and baby to car	
Nutrition	☐ Regular diet	☐ Regular diet	
Education/ Discharge Planning	☐ Sitz bath ☐ Infant care class ☐ Discharge planning ☐ Infant safety ☐ S&S of dehydration and infection ☐ Circumcision care if baby circumcized ☐ Breast pump if needed	☐ Discharge instructions ☐ Gift pack ☐ Infant car seat requirement ☐ Smoke detector ☐ Follow-up appointments ☐ Educational needs summary	☐ Reinforce teaching of infant and self–care by HHC nurse
Home Care	☐ Notify home care of delivery	☐ Home care contact in hospital	☐ Scheduled home care visits 24-48 hours post discharge
Variances *Order* *Reason* *Order* *Reason* *Order* *Reason*	☐	☐	☐ Earlier home care if needed ☐ 2nd home care visit if needed

RN Signature: _____   _____   _____
                    _____   _____   _____
                    _____   _____   _____

Confirmed post delivery by obstetrician:

_____   _____
Signature   Date

Source: Thomas Jefferson University Hospital; Women and Children Care; Philadelphia

N-1
Cesarean Delivery
Critical Pathway: Infant

Date of Birth _____   Time of Birth _____
Date of Discharge _____   Time of Discharge _____

	0-6 Hours	7-12 Hours	13-18 Hours	19-24 Hours
Laboratory/ Diagnostic Tests	Coombs Maternal Hep B status			Coombs results Maternal RPR status at delivery Bilirubin at age 24 hours PKU at age 24 hours
Treatments/ Procedures	Stabilization Baby ID Vital signs as per patient standard Weight Bath	Circumcision permit ------------------→ and circumcision Hep B permit		Circumcision care
Medications/IVs	Triple dye to cord Vitamin K Erythromycin ointment to eyes	HBIG if mother is Hep B positive or status unknown Hep B vaccine		
Consultations				
Activity	Radiant warmer until stable temp	Open crib	Open crib	Open crib
Nutrition	Breast–feeding/or Glucose H2O	Breast–feeding /or formula at least q 4 hrs	Breast–feeding /or formula at least q 4 hrs	Breast–feeding/or formula at least q 4 hrs
Assessments	Apgar at 1 and 5 minutes Gestational age Nursing assessment for VS, feeding, voiding, bonding	I + O Nursing assessment for VS, feeding, voiding, bonding	I + O Assess circumcision site	Physician assessment of body systems I + O Nursing assessment for VS, feeding, voiding, stooling, bonding
Education/ Discharge Planning	See mother pathway			
Home Care				
Variances: *Order* *Reason* *Order* *Reason*				

RN Signature: _____   _____   _____   _____
_____   _____   _____   _____
_____   _____   _____   _____

Target LOS = 72 Hours

Sex ___

	Day 2	Day 3	Within 2 Hours of Discharge	Home 24-48 Hours Post Discharge
Laboratory/ Diagnostic Tests	TA Bilirubin if > 5 at 24 hours	Bilirubin per protocol Bilirubin if > 5 at 24 hours		Bilirubin if > 5 or if baby jaundiced by home health nurse; report results to by pediatrician
Treatments/ Procedures	Circumcision care	Circumcision care		
Medications/IVs				
Consultations				
Activity	Open crib	Open crib	Open crib	
Nutrition	Breast–feeding/or formula at least q 4 hrs	Breast–feeding /or formula at least q 4 hrs	Breast–feeding /or formula at least q 4 hrs	Breast–feeding/or formula at least q 4 hrs
Assessments	I + O Nursing assessment for VS, feeding, voiding, stooling, bonding	I + O Nursing assessment for VS, feeding, voiding, stooling, bonding		HHC nurse assessment of physical environment and baby, incl VS, feeding, voiding, stooling, bonding, jaundice
Education/ Discharge Planning			Instructions to parents	
Home Care				
Variances: Order Reason				
Order Reason				

Target discharge status = Feeding well _____   Voiding & stooling adequately   Confirmed by pediatrician:
Maintaining temperature   Bonding

_____   _____
Signature   Date

Source: Thomas Jefferson University Hospital; Women and Children Care Program; Philadelphia

N-2
Cesarean Delivery
Critical Pathway: Mother

Date of Birth _____   Time of Birth _____
Date of Discharge _____   Time of Discharge _____

	Prenatal by 36 Weeks	Labor/ Delivery/ Recovery	OR Day Postpartum	Post-OP Day 1
Laboratory/ Diagnostic Tests	H + H Type and Screen Rubella RPR HBSAG	CBC MsBOS RPR		H + H or CBC Per Order RPR Results
Treatments/ Assessments		Prenatal Records in DR by 38 Weeks Assessment, Vital Signs	Post Partum/Post-OP Assessments Peri Care/Foley Care Oxygen PRN Duramorph Monitoring PRN	Post Partum/Post-OP Assessments Bed Bath with Assist Peri Care D/C Duramorph Monitoring as indicated
Medications/IVs	Prenatal Vitamins	Anesthesia per Order	PCA Pump Per Order IV with Pitocin Per Order IM Pain Meds Per Order	D/C PCA Pump D/C IV When Tolerating PO Rhogam PRN Rubella PRN PO Pain Meds
Consultations	Social Work per guideline		Social Work if Indicated	Lactation Counselor PRN Pediatrician Social Work PRN
Activity		Bedrest	Bedrest Pulmonary Hygiene	OOB as tolerated Pulmonary Hygiene
Nutrition	Appropriate Weight Gain	NPO, Ice Chips	NPO, Ice Chips	Clear Liquids
Education/ Discharge Planning	Childbirth Prep Classes Parentcraft Breast Feeding Class PRN Tour/Crit. Path Orientation Contraceptive Planning *Preparing for Your Baby's Birth at Jefferson* Select Pediatrician "Baby Talk" Video	Relaxation Technique Orient to Procedure, OR, and Recovery Room Breast Feeding	Orient to PCA Pump Orient to Unit Infant Feeding as Indicated Breast Pump if Needed	Handwashing Baby's Crib Infant Positioning, Feeding Body Mechanics for OOB and Ambulation Incision Care
Home Care	Referral to Home Care		Notify Home Care of Delivery	
Variances: *Order Reason Order Reason*				

RN Signature: _____ _____ _____ _____
_____ _____ _____ _____

Target Outcome = Demonstrates Parenting Skills
Minimal Physical Discomfort

Target Post Delivery LOS = 72 Hours

Sex ___

	Post-OP Day 2	Discharge Day Post-OP Day 3	Post-OP Day 4	Post-OP Day 5
Laboratory/ Diagnostic Tests				
Treatments/ Assessments	Post Partum/Post-OP Assessments	Post Partum/Post-OP Assessments		Follow-up Phone Call by P.P. nursing staff
Medications/IVs	PO Pain Meds Mylicon PRN Stool Softener PRN	D/C Prescriptions		
Consultations	Lactation Counselor PRN	Lactation Counseling PRN Pediatrician Social Work PRN		
Activity	Ambulation Self Care/Peri Care	Ambulation Self Care/Peri Care		
Nutrition	Progress to House Diet	House Diet		
Education/ Discharge Planning	Infant Care/Feeding Class D/C Planning Circumcision Care as indicated S&S of dehydration and infection	D/C Instructions Gift Pack Follow-Up Care Review prescription medication	Reinforce Post-Partum Education	
Home Care		Home Care Referral	Home Care Visit PRN	Home Care Visit PRN
Variances: *Order* *Reason* *Order* *Reason*				

Confirmed
Post-Delivery
by Obstetrician:

_____ _____ _____ _____

_____ _____ _____ _____

_____ _____ _____ _____

Signature _____   Date _____

Source: Thomas Jefferson University Hospital; Women and Children Care Program; Philadelphia

Glossary

ADPIE An acronym for a charting method that follows a recording sequence of assessment, diagnosis, plan, implementation, and evaluation.

Adventitious breath sounds Abnormal breath sounds.

Agency for Health Care Policy and Research (AHCPR) A component of the US Department of Health and Human Services; created by Congress to control Medicare spending by devising and promoting clinical practice guidelines.

American Nurses Association's Standards of Clinical Nursing Practice Define the nurse's role in the delivery of nursing care to a client or group of clients.

Analysis Separating or breaking up of any whole into its parts.

Assessment To gather specific information from the client and family to establish a database.

Auscultation Listening for sounds within the body, usually of thoracic or abdominal viscera, in order to detect some abnormal condition or to detect fetal heart sounds.

Bench mark A point of reference for systematic identification and implementation of best practices.

Body systems, assessment Data are collected within the framework of body systems (e.g., neurologic, cardiovascular, genitourinary).

Case management Organizes care to ensure that specific client outcomes are achieved within prescribed time frames through the use of appropriate resources.

Charting The process of making written entries about a client in the medical record.

Charting, narrative A written description of information about a client; information is recorded chronologically.

Client Refers to the individual, family, significant other, or the community.

Clinical pathway Interdisciplinary guidelines for rendering care to specific client population; designates a time line to achieve outcomes; may be called critical pathway or care map.

Clinical practice guidelines Delineate the care, course of action, or tactical plan for specific conditions.

Confidentiality Information obtained from the client, family, and other sources is kept secure and private by nurses and other health team members.

Continuum of care Matching the client's ongoing needs with the appropriate level and type of medical, health, or social service care.

Criterion (plural: **criteria**) A standard that can be used in judging; the degree of proficiency required to accomplish the end results.

Critical thinking An invisible process, a mental activity, that renders logical shape to the gathered data.

Culture and sensitivity tests Indicate the type and number of organisms present in the specimen (culture) and the antibiotics to which the organisms are susceptible (sensitivity).

Database (baseline data) Information about a client that includes a history and physical examination, laboratory, and diagnostic test results.

Data validation The comparison of data, subjective and objective, gathered from primary (client) and secondary sources (health record) with accepted normal standards and norms.

Etiology Causes of a client's health problem.

Evaluation Observed results are compared with established outcomes.

Family Individuals who are significant to the client.

Focus A method of charting that concentrates on specific problems.

Functional health patterns A topology that links assessment and human responses to actual or potential health problems.

Health A state of complete physical, mental, and social well-being, not merely the absence of disease or infirmity (World Health Organization, 1947).

Hierarchy of needs, Maslow's The arranging of human needs in order of importance; the five levels of the hierarchy are: (1) physiologic, (2) safety and security, (3) love and belonging, (4) self-esteem, and (5) self-actualization.

Human needs Physiologic or psychologic conditions that an individual must meet to achieve a state of health or well-being.

Implementation The phase of the nursing process in which the care plan is put into action.

Interdisciplinary health care team Providers representative of different disciplines who collaborate to meet the health care needs of clients.

Interdisciplinary care plan A blueprint of the care required by a client to attain identified outcomes and the role of the health care team members in providing services to meet those needs.

Interventions Specific actions that nurses and the interdisciplinary team implements to assist clients in achieving outcomes.

Interview Face-to-face encounter between the client and provider for purpose of gathering information.

Joint Commission of Accreditation of Health Care Organizations (JCAHO) An independent body that accredits health care organizations on the basis of established standards of health care.

Malpractice Failure to implement professional standards of practice; negligent treatment of a client by a health care team member.

Managed care A method of organizing the delivery of care that emphasizes communication and coordination of care among health care team members.

Medical diagnosis Identifies a disease process or pathologic condition; the diagnosis guides the therapeutic regimen.

Negligence Failure to behave in a reasonable and prudent manner; an unintentional tort (a wrong that can produce annihilation).

Norm An ideal or fixed standard; an expected standard of behavior of group members.

North American Nursing Diagnosis Association (NANDA) The professional nursing organization responsible for the approval of nursing diagnoses.

Nursing diagnosis A clinical judgment about individual, family, or community responses to actual and potential health problems and life processes. Nursing diagnoses provide the basis for selection of nursing interventions to achieve outcomes for which the nurse is accountable (NANDA, 1994).

Nursing diagnosis, actual Describes human responses to health condition or life processes that exist in an individual, family, or community. It is supported by defining characteristics (manifestations, signs, and symptoms) that cluster in patterns of related cues or inferences (NANDA, 1994a, p. 102).

Nursing diagnosis, risk Describes human responses to health conditions or life processes that may develop in a vulnerable individual, family, or community. It is supported by risk factors that contribute to increased vulnerability (NANDA, 1994a, p. 102).

Nursing diagnosis, wellness Describes human responses to levels of wellness in an individual, family, or community that have a potential for enhancement to a higher state (NANDA, 1994a, p. 102).

Nursing interventions classification The ordering or arranging of nursing activities into groups or sets on the basis of their relationships and the assigning of intervention labels to these groups.

Nursing process A systematic method of assessing human responses to health problems and developing written nursing care plans aimed at resolving the problems.

Objective data Observed or measured phenomena gathered by someone other than the client (for example, registered nurse) and presented factually.

Organizing data A cluster of similar pieces of data that represent a sequence of behavior over time.

Outcome Synonymous with client goals, objectives, expected outcomes, outcome behaviors, or short- and long-term goals; realistic, measurable goals or objectives that the client is expected to achieve.

Palpation The process of applying the hands or fingers to the external surface of the body to detect evidence of disease or abnormalities in the various organs.

Percussion The use of the examiner's fingers to tap the body lightly but sharply to determine position, size, and consistency of an underlying structure and the presence of fluid or pus in a cavity.

Physical examination The process of inspecting the body and its systems.

Population-specific health care programs Distinctive methods targeted at meeting the identified health care needs of a particular group of people.

Plan To devise a scheme for making, doing, or arranging; a detailed design or schedule.

Primary care Basic or general health care provided at the client's first contact with a health care system; the primary health provider facilitates health maintenance and therapy for illness, including consultation with specialists; health promotion and preventive care are emphasized.

Priority needs   Arranging the client's needs in order of their importance and urgency.

Problem-solving approach   A continuous systematic method of proposing solutions to health problems.

Reassessment   Gathering of specific information from the client and family and comparing the data with the initial assessment to determine the client's response to care.

Risk factors   May cause a client to be vulnerable to developing a health problem.

Same level of competent care   Clients with the same health care needs receive a comparable type of care delivered by proficient providers.

SOAP   An acronym for a charting method that follows a recording sequence of subjective data, objective data, analysis, and plan.

Standard   An accepted, rule, model, or measure; generally accepted criterion by which things of the same class are compared in order to determine quantity or excellence.

Subjective data   The client's perceptions and sensations (pain) of a health problem.

Synthesis   Putting together the parts to form a whole.

Taxonomy   An orderly classification system used in science; a systematic arrangement in groups or categories according to established criteria; an arrangement of phenomena into groups based on their relationships.

Verbs, measurable   Denote actions that can be seen, heard, or felt by the interdisciplinary team.

References

Agency for Health Care Policy and Research. (1992). *Acute Pain Management: Operative or Medical Procedures and Trauma*. DC: U. S. Department of Health and Human Services.

Agency for Health Care Policy and Research. (1994). *Management of Cancer Pain*. DC: U. S. Department of Health and Human Services.

Agency for Health Care Policy and Research. (1995). *Post-Stroke Rehabilitation*. DC: U. S. Department of Health and Human Services.

Allen, C. V. (1988). *Nursing Process Workbook*. MI: Allen.

Allen, C. V. (1990). The Art of Observation. *Nursing Times, 86*(2), 36–37.

Allen, C. V. (1990). Art in Nursing. *American Journal of Nursing, 90*(2), 34.

Allen, C. V. (1991). *Comprehending the Nursing Process*. CT: Appleton & Lange.

Allen, C. V. (1992). Motivating Registered Nurses to Change Their Behavior Toward Implementation of the Nursing Process. *Dissertations Abstracts International, 53*, n3-B:1290. (University Microfilms No. 9221308.)

American Nurses' Association. (1991). *Standards of Clinical Nursing Practice*. DC: American Nurses' Association.

American Nurses' Association. (1980). *The American Nurses' Association Social Policy Statement*. MO: American Nurses' Association.

Bates, B. (1995a). *A Guide to Clinical Thinking*. PA: Lippincott.

Bates, B., Bickley, L. S., & Hoekelman, R. A. (1995b). *Physical Examination and History Taking* (6th ed.). PA: Lippincott.

Black, H., Nolan, J., & Nolan-Haley, J. (1990). *Black's Law Dictionary* (6th ed.). MN: West.

Black, J. M., & Matassarin-Jacobs, E. (1995). *Luckmann and Sorensen Medical-Surgical Nursing* (4th ed.). PA: Saunders.

Dorland's Medical Abbreviations. (1992). PA: Saunders.

Carroll-Johnson, R. M., & Paquette, M. (1994). *Classification of Nursing Diagnoses: Proceedings of the Tenth Conference*. PA: Lippincott.

Goodman, L. S., & Gillman, A. (1990). *The Pharmacological Basis of Therapeutics* (8th ed.). NY: Pergamon.

Gordon, M. (1994). *Nursing Diagnosis: Process and Application* (3rd ed.). MO: Mosby.

Henderson, V. (1966). *The Nature of Nursing*. NY: Macmillan.

Joint Commission on Accreditation of Healthcare Organizations. (1995). *1996 Comprehensive Accreditation Manual for Hospitals*. IL: JCAHO.

Kee, J. L. (1990). *Handbook of Laboratory and Diagnostic Test with Nursing Implications*. CT: Appleton & Lange.

Kozier, B., Erb, G., Blais, K., & Wilkinson, J. (1995). *Fundamentals of Nursing* (5th ed.). CA: Addison-Wesley.

Maslow, A. H. (1968). *Toward a Psychology of Being*. (2nd ed.). NY: Van Nostrand Reinhold.

McCloskey, J. D., & Bulechek, G. M. (1992). *Nursing Interventions Classification (NIC)*. MO: Mosby.

North American Nursing Diagnosis Association. (1994). *Nursing Diagnoses: Definitions & Classification 1995–1996*. PA: NANDA.

North American Nursing Diagnosis Association. (1994). *Nursing Diagnoses: Proceedings of the Tenth Conference*. PA: Lippincott.

Orem, D. E. (1985). *Nursing: Concepts of Practice*. (3rd ed.). NY: McGraw-Hill.

Roy, C. (1984). *Introduction to Nursing: An Adaptation Model*. (2nd ed.). NJ: Prentice-Hall.

U. S. Bureau of Census. (1994). *Income, Poverty, and Valuation of Non-cash Benefits: 1993*. Washington, DC: U. S. Bureau of the Census.

INDEX

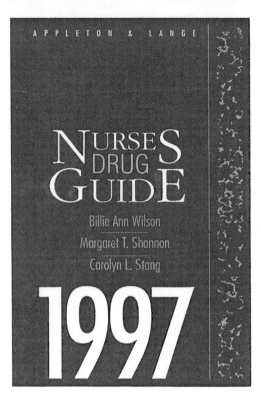